AGASTHYA
ON THE
ETERNAL CONTINUUM

AGASTHYA
ON THE
ETERNAL CONTINUUM

SURESH HARIRAMSAIT

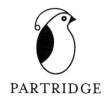

PARTRIDGE

To order additional copies of this book, contact
Partridge India
000 800 10062 62
orders.india@partridgepublishing.com

www.partridgepublishing.com/india

Contents

Preface

Rene Descartes the 16th century French psychologist and considered to be the father of modern psychology had said: *"Cogito ergo sum"* (I think therefore I am!). Only a human or a being with a highly developed state of mind can know, be aware and state that he exists. A parrot, cow, horse, elephant, chimpanzee or even a dolphin wouldn't or could not state likewise though people are now beginning to accept that various forms and species of life like the whale are *Personalities*. But is it enough for us to be aware that we exist? Don't we need to introspect further? From *where* did we come from? What now since we are here? And where do we go (after)?

'Yoga' teaches and guides us to introspect and delve deeply within ourselves to touch our core that leads us to infinite possibilities. Infinite joy, infinite knowledge and infinite expansiveness are all possibilities and are experienced just as the ancient Vedas term the Soul (our true self and the core) as 'Satchitananda' – 'Sat': Existence Absolute;'Chit': Knowledge Absolute';'Ananda': Bliss Absolute.

Immortality and infinite knowledge is already *programmed* within us (eons ago man lived for even a hundred thousand years *normally*, for the Vedas say that man was programmed to live for 100, 000 years in the first eon known as the 'Kreta yuga', 10, 000 years in the 'Treta yuga', 1000 years in the 'Dwapara yuga' and 100 years in the present one known as the 'Kali yuga').

And like Genesis in the Holy Bible says that *"there were giants on earth in those days"* and 'Hadith' another holy book of Islam says that when Adam landed on earth he was '60 cubits' or 100 feet tall, many ancient Indian texts like 'Bogar 7000' say that many eons ago man was *"as tall as a full-grown palmyra tree"* which even in present-day ideal conditions grows 50 to 60

feet tall and the Vedas further say man's *average* height was 32 feet and
he was indeed 100 feet tall!. All these could be *reprogrammed* and they
could be all 'Totally Recalled' in man through Yogic practices. Carl Jung
the pupil of Sigmund Freud says that no one is born a *'tabula rasa'*, with a
clean-slate, we all carry memories of our experiences gathered right from
the time we were single-celled protozoa and *"blocked-off memories"* have
recordings of all experiences and a *"collective unconsciousness"* of entire
mankind contains Vedic, Biblical and other ancient mythological stories
and characters that give shape to the characters in our dreams, nightmares
and inspirations.

Jonas Salk: *"At an early stage in the evolutionary process there had formed
what has been referred to as 'the thread of life' – the self-copying tape-
like molecule that contains the code which transmits to each succeeded
generation the information which, when decoded, forms the organism
prescribed in it.This code contains the 'wisdom' of previous generations of
living things..."*. *"From the moment of conception, and also at birth, each
of us is essentially a 'package of potential'."*

Many religions and philosophies of the world say that we are born sinners,
but it is the Hindu religion and Yoga that boldly state that we are *born* and
by *nature* are Perfect. Like mud covers the brilliance of a diamond or a
precious gem and soot masks the light of a lamp and hyacinth conceals the
clear-waters of a lake, three 'stains' veils our purity and divinity. Although
those stains are the cause for us taking repeated births, salvation is always
possible and eternal damnation is never an issue. Thiruvalluvar another
Tamil Siddhar who lived two thousand years ago in his 'Thirukural' states:
"Those who perform thavam (penance) create their Karma (destiny)
(*"Thavam seyvaar thum karmam seyvaar..."*); all others wallow in pain
and grief being ensnared in desires and cravings."

Just by aligning one's consciousness with the breath, at either point of
inhaling the breath or at the other end of the cycle when one exhales
completely and at that point of emptiness, one is able to touch his core when
the mind is also negated or empty. The 'Sri Shiva Sutras' say that just as
when an atom is sought and split, infinite energy is released, when the mind
is obliterated, infinite knowledge is revealed.Tirumoolar the ancient Tamil

Siddhar (Perfected Being) has in his 'Thirumandiram' stated that by stilling the mind, one is able to realize that he (*"Jivan yendru Sivan endru varellai"*) the individual Soul and 'Siva' are no different; and Saint Patanjali right in the first among his 195 'Yoga Sutras' elaborates on 'Yoga' (which derives from the Sanskrit word 'Yuj' or yoke together the soul and the Lord): *"yoga chitta vritti nirodhaha"* – "keeping the mind in an unchanged (tranquil) state is yoga"; and Osho in his 'Zero Experience' says that one should now and then delve into the state of zero experience (that the Zen masters call 'mushin' – the state of 'no-mind') to realize his true nature (and potential); and Lord Rama in the 'Rama Gita': *"Thoughtless mind is Brahman (God)"*.

The Lord Jesus Christ (in the Holy Bible, Matt:5, 48) says that we too should attain the Perfect state of the Lord and again (in Rom:8, 29) says that the *eternal plan* is to make everyone attain the exact image (replica) of the Son (Jesus) who himself is in the exact image of the Father. Hanuman in the 'Ramayana': *"As long as I am limited by my body, bound by its senses and its cravings, You are the Lord and I am your loyal servant; When 'Jivatma bodha'(knowledge of the Soul) dawns in me, I realize that You are the 'Purna' (the Whole) and I am the 'Amsa' (exact replica) of You; when 'Suddha Chaitanya bodham'(Pure Wisdom of the Soul) blossoms in me, there is absolutely no difference between You and me, I am You and You are me."*

According to Yoga we are born perfect in the *physical* also, that is apart from the nine openings present in a human adult, the new born baby has a tenth opening at the crown of the head (that is soft to the touch) which gets obliterated when we are eight to nine months old. The tenth opening is known as *'Brahmarandhara'* or the "portal or doorway of the Lord" and in English is known as 'anterior fontanelle'. And 'Prana' the dynamic energy and sum total of all forces in nature that is present in a ultra-subtle state in air enters a mystic-opening present between the upper palate of the mouth (known as *unnakku* or *annakku* in Tamil) and the brahmarandhara at the crown of the head. As long as prana enters the mystic-opening man is Perfect. Western science too says that the new born baby lives in and experiences the state of infinity until it is eight to nine months old and only after that does it become *aware* of space, individuality and body limitations. Thirumandiram 805:

"If you can send the breath twain
into the internal-tounge's upper-cavity
You shall not be bound by time;
And the gates of nectar will open be;
Graying and wrinkling will disappear
For all to see;
Youthfull will the person be
This is the Word of the Lord Nandhi."

There are 18 'evolutionary cycles' going on in 224 'bhuvanas' or global constellations in "7 upper worlds" and "7 lower worlds" containing countless universes and our (human) cycle is progressing in the lowest plane known as 'Bhuloka' in the seven upper worlds. Apart from us, there is the cycle of the 'Devas' (Angels), 'Asuras' (Titans), 'Rakshasa' (Demons), 'Kinnarva' and 'Ghandarva' (Celestial bards and dancers), 'Naga' (beings of the nether worlds having human faces with serpentine bodies etcetera. We take numerous births starting from a blade of grass to shrubs, creepers, plants, trees, birds, reptiles, animals, human, angels …, Lord Shiva in the 'Sri Shiva Rahasya' specifically says that we take 84, 000 births and 6000 births as human alone! As long as we are entrapped in the painful cycle of birth and death, we according to our degree of merits (*punya*) and de-merits (sins, *papa*) committed we either go to heaven and hell (of which there are different categories, in fact there are said to be 28 hells, that are all temporary arrangements). The Vedas even claim that there is a heaven for war-heroes as is also said in the epic 'Mahabharata' that Karna among many others entered that sort of heaven after his vanquish in the battlefield.

Yoga states emphatically that only when we realize our divinity and realize that we are not confined to the body alone, do we get out of the vicious and painful cycle of death and birth!

The three stains (*malas*) that veil our true nature are: Pride or ego (*'Anava mala'*), residues (existing as memories that could be broadly termed as 'magnetic-impurities' in the astral and subtle bodies that might also manifest as physical or mental diseases) due to good or bad acts committed in past lives (*'Kanma* or *Karma mala'*) and the Illusive-Power of the Lord that clouds our mind and make us believe that all the worlds and countless life-forms are different from the Lord (*'Maya mala'*).This concept is revealed when the Lord enlightens the four 'mind-born sons' (*manasa puthra*) of Lord Brahma the Creator: The Lord is seated under a great Banyan tree with the four Sages seated before Him and the Lord initiates them into this Wisdom through *'mauna upadesa'* (silent-communion) and by showing the 'chin mudra' (body-gesture that generates tremendous energy). His index finger folded back to touch the tip of the thumb to form a perfect circle and the other three fingers spread out that symbolizes that when one gets rid of the three primary stains, man symbolized by the index-finger and the thumb which is the Lord, merge together to become One!

One can get rid of the stains that are the cause of taking birth again and again and get physical as well as spiritual liberation by either by mingling with our Core (the Soul) which is none other than an extension of the Lord or through Yogic-means ascending with consciousness and pure awareness above the crown of the head and surrendering at the 'Holy Feet' of the Lord that is the 'Nada Bindu' the 'Eternal Sound-Light' stream of vibrations. The Lord according to the 'Saiva Siddhanta Philosophy' of the Tamils say that He is in nine forms under three categories: Form, Form-Formless and Formless. The Lord is ever present in His Formless-aspect as the 'Eternal Sound-Light Continuum' above the crown of man's head, the Yogi who with Total Awareness surrenders at the Source, is the Knower of All, is Omniscient, Omnipresent and Omnipotent.

The Holy Bible says that man was created a *"little less than god"* but Yoga says that there is absolutely no difference between the Lord and the full-blown Yogi. 'Adi Sankara' in his 'Viveka Chudamani' says that just as it is a fallacy to think that the empty space within a pot (*gada akasa*) and the space without it are two, the individual mind (within a head, be it human, cat or bird) and the Cosmic mind are not different!

People all over the world have acquired or should we say regained or recollected knowledge of arts and science or even new languages through 'Acquired Savant Syndrome'. By receiving unexpected blows to the head some in an instant have become masters of music, mathematics etcetera and some have through the 'Foreign Accent Syndrome' caused merely by the shock caused by the extraction of a tooth have started to speak in other accents and some like a person in Russia started to speak the Turkish language after getting out of a comatose-state due to a block of ice falling on his head.

But even the recollections mentioned above is not 'Total Recall'. Yoga elaborates that all worldly knowledge contained in what is known as *'Apara Vidya'*, the '64 Arts' or "branches of knowledge" is *programmed* into us. Through Yogic practices all worldly knowledge can be recollected! Even *'Para Vidya'* or 'Divine Wisdom' is programmed within. The 'Kala Tattva' or the 'Time Concept' is also programmed within which when transcended turns a person immortal and can live for as long as he desires in the physical and *leave* his body willingly with total awareness at a pre-determined time which in Sanskrit is known as *'iccha mrityu'* and the art of deathlessness in Tamil is known as *'Saha Kalai'*. Further among the '36 Tattvas' or Principle ingredients that make the finer or subtle and spiritual bodies of man, the final 5 tattvas are the 'Siva Tattvas' being the ingredients of the Primal Lord!

The *'Ashtanga Siddhis'* or the eight great Supernatural Powers come of their own accord to the Full-blown Yogi, they are "Anima, Mahima, Laghima, Garima, Prapti, Parakamyam, Vasitvam and Istvam". The Yogi hence can turn his body tinier than an atom, turn it into infinite proportions, turn it lighter than a feather, turn it heavier than a mountain, get all that he desires, teleport to distant places and enter other bodies, bring all of nature and all living-beings under his control and acquire all Powers of the Lord! Thirty-two 'minor' Powers are also attained through which he can cure incurable diseases, bring the dead back to life, turn base metal into gold, materialize and de-materialize any object including his own body, look and locate hidden treasures in the depths of the earth and oceans…!

The 'Bheranda Samhita': "*There is no greater force than maya which binds one to another, and to break that powerful bond, there is no greater force than Yoga.*"

The Lord on Yoga in the Shiva Rahasya: *"There is nothing that cannot be attained through the Power of Yoga…"* *"Yoga is the Power of Unity – the Unity between Body, Mind and Soul is of the Human kind, that which is between Man and Nature is of the Worldwide Kind, but that which is between Man and the Lord is indeed Divine".*

Acknowledgements

I had always been fascinated with Agasthya and his Super-human feats who Lord Siva equates with Himself. I've therefore based my work as a novel wherein the revered Sage Agasthya who is beyond the realms of Space and Time, clearing the doubts of two students from Wales. One is Shyam who had transited (who was my elder brother's son and had died a couple of years back in a tragic car accident in India), and the other is his (imaginary) girlfriend Heidi from Germany another country I adore for their efficient machines!

Agasthya explains to the young couple on the intricacies of life and that it is an eternal infinite continuum. The process of creation, sustenance and destruction is an never-ending one. Creation starts at the beginning or dawn of every day of the day of the Creator that lasts for 432 crore (4.32 billion years and known as a 'kalpa') and ends at dusk and the entire night-time which lasts for another 4.32 billion years as rest-time. The period of 4.32 billion years is again divided into 14 'manvantars' each lasting 308 million years or so. And then there are four cyclic-eons known as 'yugas' at the end of which there are massive catastrophes that lead to destruction. At the end of every 4.32 billion years there is deadly drought followed by relentless rain and global-level flooding and complete destruction and death of all forms of life. At dawn Creation is again resumed, but after 100 such 'Brahma or Creator-years' (8.64 x 100 billion years) all planets of the lower three 'worlds' with their countless planets, satellites and stars would all be destroyed after 100 years of drought and fire followed by 100 yeara of relentless rain and all the atoms of the worlds blowing up and everything reverting back to their original form being 'Nada Bindu'.

Agasthya explains that Creation, Sustenance and Annihilation are a sport for the Lord whose cycles are countless and finding *physical* proof would be next to impossible for all the atoms of the lower three planes containined in billions of heavenly bodies would all be blown up! He also says that it is maya which is the mighty illusive power of the Lord that veils ours as well as the true nature of all things and further expands that the Siddhars who are masters of alchemy repeatedly say that like when 'verdigris' the green rust in copper is removed lead turns into gold, when the three stains of arrogance, remanant-residues of previous births and ignorance are removed (by yogic means) man attains the Radiant-Form of the Lord!

Worlds in all (dimensions and planes - *"Ullagam yavayum"*) and in their entirety by a mere wish are being created, sustained and annihilated continuously in endless cycles and are performed effortlessly with utmost ease as if in infinite number of sports (*"Allhavilla vilayatudayan"*) by one Person, and to that One, we bow our heads (in surrender) says the 12th century Tamil Saint-Poet Kamban right in the beginning of his masterpiece 'Kamba Ramayanam'.Many luminaries even earlier had rightly presumed that life is indeed a play a game as also pointed out quite recently by the English Bard: "All the world is a stage..." ('As You Like It').

To understand a game one needs to get involved in it and to understand the Lord's play what better way is there than 'Yoga' for yoga itself is derived from the Sanskrit word 'Yuj' which means yoke, join and in its spiritual sense, it is the process by which the human spirit is brought into near and conscious communion with and is merged in the Divine Spirit. Full-blown Yogis like Thirumoolar and Adi Sankara had realized that there is absolutely no difference between the individual spirit and the Cosmic Spirit. Just as space is one regardless of it being encompassed within a pot, a house or just open space, the mind too being one whether being held within a cat or a human-head, when realization dawns, he like countless drops of rain-water that once more merges with the ocean, is once more part of the Whole.

And to surrender at the 'Holy Feet' of the Lord, the 'Purna Yogi' or Full-blown Yogi have known for eons that the Holy Feet exists as the *'Eternal Sound-Light Continuum'* (the timeless Vedas and the 'Saiva Siddhanta' philosophy of the Tamils also have pointed out specifically that one among the 'nine states' of the Lord is the 'Formless-State' of 'Nada Bindu' ('Nadha Vindhu' in Tamil), the eternal Sound-Light stream of vibrations) that exists above the crown of the head of man. When through Yogic breathing techniques and meditation one transcends from the base Chakra at the bottom of the spinal column taking along the 'Kundalini' or 'Cosmic energy', the Creative Power of the Lord that lies dormant in man (in its fiery-form as it does in the core of the earth as well as within all the heavenly bodies) with full faith and consciousness and along the upward journey, activating the other six chakras which are all energy, psychic and Wisdom-centres and finally attain the 'Eternal Sound-Light' pulses that exists even above the 'Sahasra Chakra'(or the 'thousand-petalled' Chakra) at the crown of the head, the Son and Father are One.

'**Agasthya!**'('Agasthiyar' in Tamil) the very word reverberated in Shyam's head and stirred a host of strange but wonderful emotions in his entire body, mind and soul when he first heard the name uttered by his German girlfriend Heidi and college-mate at the University of Wales, Bangor in the United Kingdom where they were both studying in their final year. A chance meeting or even hearing the name of a saint or a Perfected Being is due to karma (fate) as every happening and occurence in life too is due to past connections good or bad. Many a saint like Raghavendra who lived about four hundred years ago have mentioned that getting hold of their books (and/ or biographies) and reading them means that we had close connections and been with them personally in our past lives.

Though Shyam was an Indian and a Tamil by birth, it seemed strange for Heidi a foreigner to mention the name of Agasthya who was also an ancient Tamil speaking 'Siddhar' or Perfected Being. But right from the dawn of time both Tamil and Sanskrit had linkages with all global as well as celestial languages and cultures for it is mentioned in many ancient Indian Scriptures that the two languages and through them ancient knowledge was passed on through the ages down by celestial and other messenger-forms known as '*Deva Paramparai*' and '*Boodha Paramparai*'.

Heidi's country Germany as well as many European Cultures were always familiar with many Indian customs like the Swastika (made famous later on by Adolf Hitler and his third Reich) Fire, Sun and Nature-worship which were later discarded as 'Pagan' customs. In fact 'Agni Hothra' which is an ancient sacred Fire-worship and sacrificial-ritual is greatly respected and followed even now in Germany and in the U.S. They know that by burning cow-dung soaked in pure 'ghee' or clarified butter with a few grains of raw rice in an inverted pyramid-shaped copper-vessel the surrounding air is greatly purified, O3 is generated along with opening up of multi dimensions of space whereby various unknown rays nullify the effects of poisonous gases (and even nuclear radiation) as were proved in the recent infamous 'Bhopal gas tragedy' when thousands of people died while two families escaped the deadly onslaught because they diligently practiced the sacred ritual.

It is also a well known fact that when the famous German Sanskrit scholar Max Muller was requested by none other than Thomas Alva Edison to speak a few words over the 'radiograph' in the nineteenth century and being the first innaugural speech, he chose a Sanskrit mantra from the Rig Veda to invoke the blessings of 'Agni' the Lord of Fire, the Sun-god as well as the Creator.

Heidi had heard of Agasthya from her dad back in her home town Dusseldorf in Germany who repeatedly told her even when she was a child of many wonderful mystical stories of ancient Indian Yogis and Siddhars being super human beings and about their incredible deeds. Her little eyes had expanded in wonder when her dad had told her that those men and women by controlling Prana which was the life-force and sum total of all forces in nature within their bodies, had control of the infinite Prana *outside* too and thus had control over entire nature. By gaining control over Prana they even defied death and could live for as long as they wanted. They also avoided the agonizing cycle of birth and death for only when man dies an 'unconscious' death does re-birth take place. The death of a Perfected Being is an entirely conscious one performed with total awareness by forcing the life-force to gently ascend through the *'Brahmarandhara'* or "the gateway of the Lord" being the 'tenth opening' at the crown of the head.

Heidi's dad Karl oft repeated stories of the Siddhars of India and his father's brief glimpse of the venerated sage Agasthya at the foothills of the 'Pothigai' or Agasthya mountain as is also known had kindled within her the spirit and later rage to visit the holy places spread out among the Himalayan ranges and mountains at the southern tip of India. Karl's father Gustav had along with a couple of Europeans and an American girl in July 1937 just pitched their tents at dusk besides a large pool (right at the base of the 'Pothigai Mountain') of sweet water known as *'Poonkulam'* or literally "the lake of flowers" which indeed it was for its banks and sandy beaches were bordered with bush and creepers enveloped with sweet-smelling jasmine and other exotic flowers. The pool was also the source of the Tamiraparani river which flew down to Papanasam about fifteen miles downstream and finally merged with the ocean waters of the Bay of Bengal fifty miles to the east.

Gustav along with Jane the American had strolled a couple of miles to the east and unknowing had stumbled accidently upon a place known as 'Sangumuthirai' or the 'Conch-seal' stamped on a large rock which lay directly on the foot-path at the base of the Pothigai mountain and led right to the summit that was six thousand one hundred and odd feet high. Just as they decided to turn back to camp for it was starting to turn dark rapidly as it always does as people accustomed to Indian forests and jungles know, they saw a sight which was to be firmly entrenched in their minds for the rest of their lives and maybe even beyond. At a distance of a hundred yards or so they saw twenty one huge elevated rocks on a plain ground which were actually holy altars and on them were seven radiant beings seated in a semi-circular manner besides seven sacrificial fire-pits, offering flowers, holy twigs and ghee-soaked grains to the Holy-Fire and at the same chanting Vedic-Mantras which they could distinctly hear. When they attempted to get closer they were held back by some unseen force and what was more terrifying was the sudden burst of trumpet sounds, crack of bamboo trees snapping and undergrowth being trampled upon by huge beasts and occasionally squealing noises which all heralded the approach of a large herd of wild elephants. Gustav and Jane froze in their tracks for they knew it was certain death if they were caught out in the open with thirsty baby, mother and bull elephants that were hurrying to bathe and quench their thirst in their regular water-hole before turning dark. Luckily they were placed downwind so they made a hasty retreat.

Only when they were back in camp did it strike in Gustav's mind the significance of the sight they had just witnessed for in an instant he knew that the seven holy radiant-beings they had seen were none other than the 'Saptha Rishis' or seven celestial messengers often mentioned reverentially in various ancient Indian texts! Gustav had read that the seven seers closely monitored entire creation and that he was indeed blessed and fortunate to have a glimpse of them (for they could remain unseen if and when needed for they were beyond the realms of space and time) with a certain purpose and to perhaps remind man now and again that Superior forces were watching and guiding him.

Karl had also been fortunate to have a passing glimpse of the seer Agasthya more than three decades later when he was with a couple of European tourists. Karl like his dad earlier had gone for a stroll all alone at the base of the Pothigai Mountain similarly at dusk and was in a shola which is a thick jungle covered with a canopy made of gigantic trees. Even as it was getting quickly dark, he saw something glimmer at a distance within the confines of the leafy jungle and he stopped to concentrate better. Ahead at a distance of roughly hundred feet or so he saw a short-statured bearded radiant-being crossing his path. When he had a clearer view, he could see that the figure had a halo that was golden-yellow in color, seemed to glide above the earth and he had such a tremendous magnetic-pull that dried leaves that littered the ground floated behind him for a distance before falling back to earth. Karl could see even the dried leaves shimmering in the proximity of the radiance that emitted from the seer. When karl reached the exact spot where the seer had crossed his path he could see that the dry leaves on the ground still retained some of the glow which slowly faded out. When Karl tried to call out to the quickly disappearing figure, to his surprise nothing emanated from his mouth and all that he remembered was the seer as he later learnt chanting 'Siva Siva' as he glided ahead with what seemed to be closed eyes!

Shyam like Heidi *knew* in the deepest recesses of his mind and soul that he was destined to meet the holy Seer Agasthya. Both of them had with eagerness planned to travel to India during their upcoming winter holidays, go to the Pothigai hills (as the group of mountains in the Papanasam and Courtallam area were generally known), climb up to the summit of the 'Agasthya malai' named after the holy Seer himself and somehow meet the Sage. Though Shyam was never inclined to turn towards any sort of religion, cult or Yoga, nor was he an atheist, through his dad he had come to know that he was born a *Namboodhiri* in the neighboring state of Kerala in his previous life and so spiritualism was deeply ingrained within him. Namboodhiris like some sects of the Jews are very religious and orthodox people and some of them even have been nurturing the flames of ritual Sacrifical sacred Fire of the Vedic times for thousands of years within their homes. Shyam's family for generations were very wealthy traders settled in the vicinity of the Pothigai hills in a town on the banks of the Tamiraparani river in the state of Tamilnadu, but a couple of centuries back had migrated from the state of Kerala lying on the Arabian sea coast.

Shyam's dad Soke had with doubts sent along the palm imprints of his son's right-hand on a sheet of paper through a friend who in turn had sent it through another friend to prophecy his son's immediate future and his past life to the 'Vaidheeswaran Temple' in a very ancient town Kumbakonam in Tanjore district of Tamil Nadu. There are many astrologers who read and interpret palm-leaf manuscripts which are matched against a person's palm-imprints, but the ones at this particular temple-town and especially the one who was sought after was an honest person who read and interpreted palm-leaf manuscripts written in Tamil by the ancient Ramayana era sage 'Vasishta'.

The messenger who bore Shyam's palm-imprints knew nothing of him or his family nor was anything mentioned to him for him to intentionally or un-intentionally give away details. The main astrologer was an aged person with very poor eyesight so his trained son read-out the Tamil inscriptions while his father interpreted them and another assistant wrote them down and in the same time recorded the same on a cassette. The person who went for the prophecy could question the astrologer on thirteen 'Kandams' or subjects like past-life, present-life, family-life, names of family members, business- status, future-life if any etcetera. The money charged for the prophecy too was meager and cost only a couple of hundred rupees.

When Shyam along with his dad and mom heard the prophecy they were astounded for every detail of his life was explained in detail. Shyam's and his younger sister's name was give along with his dad's and mom's and what was even more amazing was even his future wife's town and children's names were given. The icing on the cake was when it was clearly mentioned that Shyam was born as a Namboodhiri in his past life in a town known as 'Guruvayur' famous for its Lord Krishna Temple in the state of Kerala. Shyam's dad Soke immediately reminded them that this could be true for their family lineage-name was 'Thambaradiyan' and as the name suggested their fore-fathers had played the 'thambra' or drums during the ancient Guruvayur Lord Krishna Temple's flag-hoisting and other temple festivals! The Thambaradiyan people had two centuries or so earlier migrated from

Guruvayur on the western-side of the Pothigai hills to a beautiful place along the banks of the Tamiraparani river on the eastern-side of the holy hills. The place they selected to settle down was in the confluence of three rivers: the Tamiraparani, Manimutharu river and the Rama river and hence later became known as 'Mukkudal'(three confluences).

It was therefore not surprising that strange and wonderful emotions stirred within Shyam when the name 'Agasthya' was uttered in his presence. Further Shyam's great-grandfather who had been a pious and holy man had once met a Siddhar in Papanasam below the Pothigai hills who after studying his breathing-pattern told him that he was of the lineage of the great Seer and Siddhar Agasthya.When questioned the Siddhar replied that all human beings could be classified under the lineage of the 'eighteen Primary Siddhars' (the eighteen most important siddhars among a host of others) and his breathing-pattern was that of Agasthya.

Shyam's prophecy also mentioned that though being a Priest and devotional person in his previous life, he after murdering his wife fled away with an younger beautiful girl after looting the jewels and vast riches of the holy temple in which he was until then conducting pujas (prayer rituals). But as mentioned by Lord Krishna in the Bhagavad Gita, a person who practises Yoga and its tenets with devotion and discards it mid-way, is born again in a pious or rich family and once more proceeds from where he had left it in his previous life, Shyam once again proceeded to start his life of Yoga and devotion triggered by a what seemed to be chance hearing of the name 'Agasthya'.

Shyam and Heidi after taking the train-ride to London from Bangor in Wales, boarded the immediate British Airways flight to New Delhi. The six feet three inches tall Shyam and Six footer Heidi did not look like an odd couple for many students, friends and working partners from right across the globe were constantly travelling to and fro from Delhi. Though Heidi looked very much the Anglo-Saxon with her blonde hair and blue eyes, Shyam looked more Latin American perhaps Brazilian with his curly hair, honey-colored texture and tall thin wiry-body.

The couple had planned to first take the famous 'Kailash Manasoravar Pilgrimage' a vital at least once in a lifetime pilgrimage for 'Saivaites' or the ones who worshipped Lord Shiva and considered Him to be the Primal Lord. Mount Kailash was more than twenty thousand feet high while Lake Manasoravar at its base was the highest fresh-water lake in the world placed at the base of the revered mountain but at a height of around fifteen thousand feet or so, about three hundred feet in depth and nestled in the Himalayas. Mount Kailash is considered to be the shadow and replica of Mount Meru in 'Kailash' being the realm of Lord Shiva Himself and the uppermost heaven among the *"seven upper and seven lower worlds"* spread across various planes and dimensions.

Shyam and Heidi had also wanted to travel further into unknown and uncharted areas of the Himalayas, especially to a highly secretive place known as *Siddhashram* situated a hundred miles or so north-east of Mount Kailash. Many 'Purna Yogis' or full-blown-Yogis who had through self-realization conquered death were said be living in that peaceful area spending a life of bliss-full meditation in either their physical or astral bodies. They had also hoped to have a chance encounter with 'Mahavatar Babaji' who is said to be more than two thousand years old, had met the Lord Jesus Christ and another Perfected Being 'Adi Sankara'. Babaji as he is more commonly known is said to roam about in the higher reaches of the Himalayas along with a few followers some of them being Americans. What interested both Heidi and Shyam was when they heard that Babaji like many full-blown Yogis was 'forever' youthful and looked not a day beyond twenty one years! They had hoped to get personally initiated into 'Kriya Yoga' and thus attain enlightenment and perhaps even the state of 'deathlessness'.

Thiruvannamalai – "as old as the Himalayas"; 'Ramana' and many Siddhars; 'Swan Craft' & 'Boar Craft'; its mountain-cave containing 'Heavenly Treasures'

All plans went astray as an avalanche swept away many pilgrims on the way up to Mount Kailash and though there were helicopter rides, even they were cancelled due to very harsh climatic conditions. Shyam after informing his dad and mom about their change of plans flew down to Chennai from New Delhi and proceeded by car along with Heidi after a night's stay to Thiruvannamalai. Thiruvannamalai with its Mount Arunachala is said to be as old as Mother Earth itself for 'Arunachala Mahimai' a holy book that glorifies the ancient hill states that even as the earth was going through spasms of birth pangs (one among many cyclic-births) and the Himalayas rose to its heights, bits were flung into the atmosphere and one of the *small* pieces landed more than thousand five hundred miles to the south which now stands a little more than two thousand feet high with a base measuring seven miles or so in circumference as Mount Arunachala.

The Lord Shiva Temple at Thiruvannamalai is considered to be one of the holiest and ancient ones in India. Even if a person even just *thinks* about it, one would be absolved of his sins and attain *'Mukti'* (liberation and take no more births and put an end to the misery-filled endless cycle of death and birth) whereas one needs to be *born* in Madurai and *die* in Kasi or Benares to attain the same.

Another incident stated in many ancient Puranas like the 'Linga Purana' swears on its antiquity. When two among the Holy Trinity Lord Brahma the Creator and Lord Vishnu the Sustainer argued on who was the greater among them, there appeared an infinite column of light between them. Lord

Brahma to seek its source took to flight in his 'Anna Vahana' or 'Swan Craft' and soared and flew even beyond the "seven upper worlds", Lord Vishnu in his 'Varaha Vahana' or 'Boar Craft' *tunnelled'* his way through the "seven lower worlds" and went even beyond 'Baathala', 'Kanniktai' and 'the twenty-eight hells'. Neither of them could find the beginning and end of the infinite pillar of Light. Only after accepting defeat, did a voice call out from the column of Light stating that He Lord Shiva had appeared in that infinite-form above and below the holy Arunachala Mountain!

The Sthala Puranam that bears the history of the holy temple says that there would always be a couple of Purna or full-blown Yogis in the vicinity of the temple for all ages to come. Recent yogis who lived there were Seshadri swami, Sri Ramana Maharishi and Yogi Ramsuratkumar who all attracted hosts of devotees the most famous of them being Paul Brunton of the U.S.. The latter's many doubts were cleared just by sitting before the tranquil presence of Sri Ramana and according to Brunton himself the peace generated by the yogi was found nowhere else in the world.

Regarding Yogi Ramsuratkumar, Shyam recollected what his paternal uncle Suresh had told him. Exactly three decades earlier Suresh at the age of twenty-seven who was an atheist at that time, had along with a few friends met the Yogi.The Yogi who immediately sensed that the lad had come with a lot of doubts and misgivings, seated him beside him, held his hands in his lap and smiled at him with both warmth and mirth.When he suddenly blurted out: *"This fellow Suresh thinks I am mad!"* Suresh was shocked, for that was what he was thinking at the moment! The yogi then without being questioned, said: *"Yes! There are people out in the stars!"* This was also right for Suresh was bursting to ask about aliens! Suresh was then floored when the yogi requested a girl to fetch him a spoon and served him a sweet using it only for him whereas all others were served right out of his hand (Suresh had been thinking with dread on how he was going to accept the sweet served by the yogi whose hands and nails looked filthy and were filled with dirt!).

Shyam and Heidi after checking into a hotel went to the Thiruvannamalai Temple to pray to Lord Shiva and the Holy Mother. The temple bore scores of stories of yogis who had appeared and vanished all of a sudden and the couple had even seen on 'Youtube' of a sitting yogi suddenly flying and vanishing into space; of Seshadri Swami bringing a dead horse back to life and of the real death of a lad who tried to fool the yogi of a fake death!; about the 10th century Saint Arunagiri who was saved by the Lord Himself after he jumped off from the heights of the temple tower and after singing thousands of chaste Tamil songs turned himself into a parrot and is still believed to be living in that form as of date!

They later went to the Ashram of Sri Ramana which still possesses an immense aura radiating peace and tranquility that emanates from the Samadhi or tomb of the Maharishi. Though Sri Ramana attained the exalted state of *'Jivan Mukti'* or liberation even while living in the physical and *'Jiva Samadhi'* – leaving the physical consciously and with total awareness in 1950 itself (and people had witnessed yogi rising up to the skies in a radiant-form) Heidi and Shyam could feel the yogi's presence and enjoyed waves of joy and what seemed to be heavenly-bliss.

Heidi's dad had told her about the discovery and sighting of heavenly treasures in a secret hidden cave in the holy mountain by Sri Ramana. Once when the yogi was in deep contemplation an abnormally large golden-colored Peepal (the 'Bodhi tree' under which Lord Buddha attained Enlightenment) tree leaf appeared on his lap and even while wondering on from where such a wonderful specimen had originated, there appeared a light. Following the light which led him to a secret hidden cave in the mountain, upon entering it, Sri Ramana found heaps and heaps of gold and priceless gems, stones and jewels. Realizing instantly that the treasures could be only of heavenly origin the yogi who himself was beyond likes and dis-likes, who regarded mud and gold, stone and diamond as one, left them un-disturbed and went back to the ashram.

And Heidi along with Shyam at dusk on that day out of curiosity walked in the particular direction from the ashram as the yogi himself had done. As light quickly vanished and there was moon-light and though they had rechargeable torches after arriving at a particular spot both of them felt giddy, swooned and fell down to the ground. Even as they recovered their composure after several minutes, they could not see anything for moon-light was blanked out in clouds and both their torches failed to function. After hearing their cries of help a sheperd approached them and led them back to safety.

Only later did they learn that more than seventy years back a few devotees of Sri Ramana had gone through a remarkably similar experience. In the late 1940's, one day when Sri Ramana had told his devotees about his discovery of heavenly treasures and the yogi had retired to his chambers at night, a couple of his inquisitive devotees gathered courage and went on a treasure-hunt. Though the yogi had warned none of them to go in the particular direction and trail that he had traversed earlier, greed and curiosity overcame them. All went fine till the trail they followed led them to the base of the mountain. When they reached a particular spot, they all turned blind, felt giddy, swooned and fell down. Recovering after some time, they shouted out in help and it was none other than the yogi himself who came to their rescue. After restoring their sight and leading them back to the ashram, he scolded them and requested them to never again to go against faith

Heidi reminded Shyam that her dad had told her many years back that whenever she had a chance to visit ancient holy temples, holy hills and particularly holy shrines that contained the Samadhis of Yogis she should be careful in respecting the laws and customs practiced by the devotees.

Samadhis were different from shrines that held the mortal remains of saints and/or divine personalities. A full-blown Yogi who is a 'realized' or 'enlightened' person would also be one who had attained *'Jiva mukti'* or one who had attained both physical and spiritual liberation (end from the endless cycle of death and birth) even while living in the physical. Such a person would often select the exact time and place where he preferred to enter into Samadhi many months or even years earlier. Instructions would be given on the dimensions of the tomb, quantity and variety of holy fragrant-materials to be placed inside and even the direction it faced. At the exact time that the Perfected Being had predicted, he or she would enter the tomb after settling any outstanding dues and duly blessing the devotees present there, sit in the 'Padmasana' (lotus-posture) facing usually the north(facing the holy Mount Kailash in the Himalayas) or north-east, with sheer force of will and along with Prana and with total awareness depart from the body through the

'*Brahmarandhara*' being the "gateway of the Lord" and the tenth-opening at the crown of the head.

Heidi's dad had learnt through many a saint in India that all such ancient temples and holy mountains that had secret hidden caves that held sealed samadhis of Perfected Beings were portals to higher and lower planes in other dimensions. The body of a Yogi would remain fresh and be preserved for eons to come and if and when needed he himself or another yogi could re-enter the body and be a guide and enhance the life of mankind. Saint Thirumoolar had after pitying the state of grieving cows entered the body of their shepherd named 'Moolan' and completed that life in the body of the shepherd after not being able to trace his own body which he had hidden in some thick bushes; Adi Sankara after asking his devotees to carefully guard his own body in a secret place had entered the body of a dead king to personally experience the life of a family-man while he himself was a hermit leading the life of a recluse!; Little is known of Shirdi Sai Baba's origin and it is said that he had entered the body of the perfectly preserved body of an Islamic saint.

Heidi and Shyam had left Thiruvannamalai after circumambulating the holy Arunachala hill which is a 13 kilometer walking trek in a somber-mood but wiser with the knowledge that one should yearn only for peace and happiness and not scamper after anything material beyond their needs.

Srirangam – "Boologa Vaikuntam" ("Ultimate Heaven on earth"); sighting of the extinct five-headed cobra; Perfectly preserved Pristine body of saint Ramanujar exactly a thousand years old; the golden Vimana (Chariot of the Lord) thousands of billions of years old; Secret chambers holding unlimited treasures

Srirangam the holy Temple of Lord Vishnu that lay between the rivers Kaveri and Kollidam near Trichy was the next destination. The young couple from the United Kingdom had heard that Srirangam was considered to be 'Boolaga Vaikuntam' or literally "Ultimate Heaven on earth" and the most important among the '108 Divya Desas' or the 108 Holy Zones of the Lord Vishnu or Narayana.

While Shyam entered the Holy Temple, Heidi walked around the outer wall ('Velhi parikaram') as people of other faiths were not allowed inside. Though several French, Italian and other foreigners stood outside the main entrance clicking away on their cameras and mobiles, Heidi's interest lay elsewhere. About a decade back a group of twenty to thirty devotees had to their amazement seen a huge five-headed cobra with all its five hoods spread-out slither gracefully in front of them and vanishing into the outer wall of the Temple. Heidi headed in that direction and stood before what she presumed to be the exact spot where the reptile was seen. Though she could see no traces of a crack or opening on the surface of the huge wall, Heidi suspected that a portal leading to other dimensions of space could have opened to allow passage of the snake and closed again for it was considered to be a close companion and 'seat' of the Lord.

Shyam on the other hand prayed at the inner 'Sanctum Sanctorium' from where 'Andal' had disappeared right before the gaze of hundreds of onlookers that included her dad 'Periazhwar'. Devotees had seen her turn into a radiant form of light and merge with the holy statue of the Lord. Shyam then had the greatest fortune of witnessing the ritual of bathing the holy body of Saint Ramanujar who had attained the Samadhi-state exactly thousand years ago. The Saint's body had turned hard as rock over the years, but it was still with great reverence bathed in medicated oil once a year, after performing pujas it was once again closed to any public view.

The couple then had a good look at the massive but beautiful golden 'Vimana' (replica of the flying-craft or chariot of the Lord which almost all temples have adorning the 'Gopuram' (tower or rounded-dome being the top or crown of the temple). The vimana as well as the statue of the Lord were even older than the earth itself for it is said that they were worshipped by the ancestors of the *'Raghu Vamsa'* or the clan in which Lord Rama was born which itself was several hundred thousand years ago, before then they adorned 'Sathya Loka' the realm of Lord Brahma the Creator for a few 'yugas'(eons) and even before that they adorned *'Par Kadal'* or the 'Ocean of milk' for many yugas and before that *'Vaikuntha'*(the realm of Lord Vishnu) itself for ages, so they were literally tens or hundreds or even thousands of billions of years old!

Before leaving for Palani, the couple also stood before locked rooms behind and underneath which existed secret hidden chambers rumored to contain treasures of incredible magnitude. The Kings and Emperors of lore had donated to many of the ancient temples gold, diamonds, rubies, precious stones and jewelry "equal to the weight of full-grown elephants". It is mentioned in stone inscriptions that Kings had two huge boats lashed together with strong wooden planks between them, floated them in the deep-waters of the Kaveri river and while in one boat stood a massive elephant the other boat was heaped with gold and invaluable precious stones equivalent in weight to the animal. Two of the most important holy Temples to which such huge periodic offerings were made are the Srirangam Temple and the other being the holy 'Padmanabasamy Temple' in Thiruvanthapuram, Kerala whose vast hidden riches were discovered only a couple of years ago and is now considered to be "the richest temple in the world."

Palani – Bogar's Samadhi; Bogar (who flew to China) and Lao Tzu one and the same;

Palani is a small rock mountain standing thousand five hundred feet tall and contains the holy Temple of Lord Muruga or Karthikeya and/or Skanda as he is known in north India. Muruga is the second son of the Primal Lord Shiva, the other being Lord Ganesha or Vinayaka the elephant-headed one. Eons ago in 'Kailash' the realm of Shiva, the primal Lord was presented the "fruit of Wisdom" by the Celestial Sage Narada (while some texts say it is a mango, others emphatically state that it is the pomegranate) which when partaken would also prove to be an ambrosia, an elixir that would provide eternal youth. While the Lord and the Divine Mother refused to partake it, there arose a contest among the two sons on whom was to be presented with the fruit of Wisdom. The contest that was decided was a race as to who was the first to circumvent the "seven upper and seven lower worlds" that contained infinite number of universes.

While Lord Muruga piloted his 'Peacock Craft' (*Mayil Vahanam*) and circumvented all the universes and entire space within a micro-second, Lord Vinayaka even before that circumvented the Divine Father and Mother who truly contained within them everything and duly claimed the prize. The enraged Lord Muruga shunned his home and his parents, flew down to earth and settled down in Palani and is there ever since blessing his devotees and his Creation being also his favorite language Tamil.

Shyam and Heidi drove down from Srirangam to Palani which was at a distance of a little more than a hundred kilometers. After refreshing themselves in a hotel, they immediately went and prayed at the holy Temple at the base of the Palani hill and then climbed up the gentle pathway that was laid in such a way as to facilitate the temple elephant to easily ascend and descend the hill. Although there was a rope-car for devotees to be ferried up the hill, the couple preferred to walk to take in the fresh cool air and study their surroundings.

At the summit's holy temple the couple went at first inside to pray before the sacred statue of Lord Muruga and requested the priest to lead them to the original 'Navabhashanam' statue of the Lord created by the venerated Sage and Siddhar 'Bogar'(Bhogar). The priest was not surprised that foreigners were aware about the presence of the original statue for there were many websites on the internet that had immense material regarding the medicinal value of the Navabhashanam or the *"nine mixtures or alloys of herbs, arsenic-like poisons and metals"*.

The priest after getting prior permission from the necessary officials led the couple to the back where stood the wonderful Navabhashanam statue of the Lord. They could see as they had read and personally heard that the statue had worn down in size through the ages due to being constantly consecrated or bathed with varied holy substances. Heidi knew through her dad and grand-dad that the surrounding air gets ionized when 'Agni Hothra' is performed, in a similar manner, scientific research had revealed that when 'Abishekam' or consecration is perfomed when alkaline products like milk, honey, sandal-paste, curd, holy-ash etcetera are poured over the statue and when camphor is lit, ionization takes place and O3 is generated in large quantities which is beneficial to all forms of life. And even beyond that the liquid collected at the base of the statue after the consecration is completed proves to be of immense curative value. Moreover greedy priests over the ages had scraped away portions of the holy statue and sold them off to traditional doctors leading to quick degradation of the statue.

After collecting some sandal-paste that was utilized in coating the Navabhashanam statue (the holy ritual known as 'Sandhana Kappu' or 'Sandal Protection') which was a very good and potent skin and body protective lotion, they went to the adjacent Samadhi of the holy Siddhar 'Bogar'.

Bogar was a full-blown Yogi who had attained the *'Ashtanga Siddhis'* or 'Eight great Supernatural Powers' and had thus travelled to and fro between

India and China (as mentioned in the sixth song of 'Bogar 7000') 'through space' (*'Ahaya Margam'*) as mentioned often by various other Siddhars, the most important among them being his disciple 'Pulipani'.

Bogar is said to have lived in the physical in 3500 B.C. at around the same period as that of 'Lao Tse'(or 'Lao Tzu') and he and Lao Tzu are said to be one and the same. Bogar's Guru or Master 'Kalanginathar' is said to be of Chinese origin who came to India and attained Samadhi here. Taoism that was founded by Lao Tzu and 'Siddha Yoga' have many things in common among them is the same principles of 'Yin' and 'Yang' and the 'Siva' 'Shakthi' – the male and female aspect. Bogar is also said to have constructed and flew aircrafts (Vimanas) to China and taught the Chinese to power and propel ships by utilizing steam by vaporizing water. Lao Tzu too like many Siddhars and Yogis of India would remain quiet and sit in a tranquil-state and to any questions of life would simply write on the river-sands: 'MEDITATE'.

After walking down the Palani hill, Shyam and Heidi once more prayed at the Temple at the base and with reverence silently prayed for the blessings of many Siddhars who are said to be in the Samadhi-state in various secret blocked-off caves deep within the hill and left for Madurai further south.

Madurai – "Primal Heaven on earth" (*'Boolokha Sivalokham'*); The "Golden-Lotus Pond" even pre-dates the rivers Ganges and Kaveri; Agasthya explains the 64 'Lilas' or 64 Divine Sports played by the Lord in Madurai; 'Iravatham' the White Elephant of Indra the Lord of the Angels cursed to be born on earth and Salvation by bathing in the holy pond

The Madurai Meenakshi Amman Temple's Sivalinga and its 'Golden-Lotus Pond' (*'Porthamarai Kulam'*) are said to be the oldest and foremost ones in not just the earth but in the seven upper and seven lower worlds. The Golden-lotus pond dates back to even before the creation of the holy river Ganges and Kaveri according to the holy Sage Agasthya himself. Agasthya mentions this fact in the introduction to the 'Thiruvilayadal Puranam' that explains the sixty four 'Lilas' or 'Divine Sports' played by the Lord Himself in person in the city of Madurai.

Heidi and Shyam after resting a bit in the 'D.T.D.C.'('Tamilnadu Tourist Development Corportion') hotel and refreshing themselves immediately went to the Holy Temple's 'Golden-lotus pond' to take a dip – a cleansing bath and let their guide explain to them in detail and lead them through the Temple.

They were blessed and fortunate enough to get such an exemplary person as 'Thilagavathy Rajasekar' to be their guide for she was an expert (and author of the 'Thiruvilayadal Puranam' in modern simple Tamil), scholar and devotee of the Lord as well as an ardent devotee of the Siddhar of Thiruvannamalai Sri Ramsuratkumar as well as the living-Saint Sri Muralidhara Swami who in fact released her book in 1986.

Thilagavathy explained to them in brief about the greatness of the Thiruvilayadal Puranam and the temple's antiquity and said that even the first 'Padalam' or chapter of the Purana begins in 'Indralokha' or heaven being the realm of Lord Indra the Lord of the 'Devas' or 'Angels' and ends at the very spot they now stood. Indra was returning to heaven after winning a battle over the 'Asuras' or 'Titans' and he was filled with pride and with great pomp was majestically riding the heavenly single-tusked white elephant 'Iravatham'. Even as he was entering his capital city 'Amaravathy' surrounded by his four types of troops (foot-soldiers, horse-mounted, chariots and elephant-mounted soldiers), the Divine-Sage 'Dhurvasa' in the midst of the mighty rich and famous presented with piety and humility to Indra a golden-lotus flower that had ordained the head of the Shivalinga of Kashi (Benares).

Indra received the offered flower with scant respect in one hand and placed it carelessly on the head of his mount Iravatham. Iravatham without a care in the world grasped the flower in its trunk, threw it down and stamped it into the ground! The enraged Sage Dhurvasa cursed Iravatham to be born on earth as a wild elephant and Indra the Lord of the Angels to be slaughtered by a Pandyan King in Madurai.

Iravatham lost its sheen, complexion and beauty and was born among wild elephants on earth. After leading a hard life among harsh conditions for a hundred years here on earth it had total recall of its past glorious life only after accidently sighting the 'Golden-lotus Pond' of the Madurai Temple. Iravatham started to perform puja (worship) at the holy Temple and would draw pure fresh water into its trunk, bathe the Shivalingam and adorn it with flowers with love and devotion. The Lord pleased by the elephants kindness and devotion, provided the wishes and boons it desired and gave it liberation. Thilagavathy thus explained to them about the greatness and holiness of the holy pond.

A heavenly "glowing light-filled Vimana" sighted with the Lord seated within; Formation of Madurai city in a 'Kadamba' tree-filled forest; 'Madhu' or elixir being the "fountain of youth" spilled out of compassion from the Crescent-moon adorning the forehead of the Lord fell on the city and thus came to be known as 'Madurai'.

Tens of thousands of years ago during the reign of Kulasekara Pandyan of the Pandyan dynasty whose capital city was known as 'Manavoor' which lay east of a huge Kadamba tree filled forest. At that time there lived a kind-hearted trader named Dhananjeyan who was greatly devoted to Lord Siva and performed many pujas, charities and other noble deeds all in the Lord's name.

One day Dhananjeyan travelled westwards and after completing trading was returning back by foot to his town of Manavoor when he had to cross the huge kadamba-forest. Even while he was crossing the forest it started to grow dark and the trader was disturbed and afraid of the consequences of a chance meeting with the many fierce wild animals that inhabited and roamed the thick undergrowth. With trepidation he walked on trying at the same time to find a possible shelter for the night when he saw a strange but wonderful soothing glowing light a little ahead among the trees and bushes. As Dhanjeyan cautiously approached the source of light, he saw with wonderment a glowing heavenly 'Indravimana' (literally a magical flying craft of the gods) radiating soothing light and observed with great joy the Grace-filled, compassionate Light-radiating Lord Siva seated within!

As it was a very holy and auspicious day, all the 'Devas' or Angels were assembled there and were praying and performing pujas directly in Person to the Lord. Dhanjeyan as luck and fate deemed it, had lots of high quality perfumes and other holy articles like 'Athar'(a highly-valued perfume) sandal-oil, turmeric, camphor, sandal-paste etcetera with him which he presented to the holy devas that were therefore utilized in the puja worship. The whole night was spent in such a way and everyone was revelling in the ecstatic-joy that was ever present in the vicinity of the Lord. Even as dawn started to break all of a sudden all the Devas had vanished with only Dhananjeyan present before the Lord. After circumambulating the Lord many times with hands raised above his head in prayer with tears of joy streaming down his face, Dhananjeya with great reluctance left the Lord to return home.

Dhanjeyan immediately went to the palace met the King and reported with great joy the sighting of the Lord and the performance of continuous prayers and pujas by all the devas for the entire night. That very night the Lord appeared in the dream of the King and asked him to clear the kadamba forest and raise a beautiful city filled with many temples containing innumerable sacrificial-altars and divine ponds. The Lord repeatedly appeared in the King's dreams as a Siddhar and guided him on how he was to lay the various tracks, roads, temples and towers in the leveled land and thus creating a beautiful city.

After completion of the city even as the King was contemplating on how he was to seek Salvation from the sins acquired by cutting down innumerable living-trees and dislocating multitudes of varying life-forms, the Lord out of compassion spilled 'madhu' (ambrosia or elixir the food of the gods) from the crescent-moon adorning his forehead that flowed all over the city and thus came to be known as 'Madurai'.

After explaining to Heidi and Shyam about the greatness and holiness of Madurai, Thilagavathy went on to show the couple the place in the holy temple the particular place where the Holy Mother Herself appeared out of a Sacrifical-Fire as a beautiful three year-old girl.

The Holy Mother appears out of a great Sacrifical-Fire as a three year-old girl;

King Kulasekara Pandyan was a very just-ruler who performed many Sacrifical-rites, pujas and provided food, clothing gold and many material articles to the poor and needy. Though the Pandyan kingdom under Kulasekaran flourished and became the foremost among the eighteen kingdoms of the then southern India, the King in due time was overjoyed when a son was born who was to be the heir to the throne and named him 'Malayathuvasa Pandyan'. After several years of just-rule a flourishing Pandyan kingdom had reached wide fame and name, King Kulasekaran performed many 'Siva-pujas' and finally de-materialized within the holy temple and attained 'Oneness' with the Lord.

King Malayathuvasa Pandyan also was a great and noble king and had many riches, was as handsome as 'Manmathan' the Lord of Love ('Cupid') and though he had ten thousand queens, his regent-queen was 'Kanchanamalai' the daughter of the King of the Chola Dynasty 'Soorasenan'. Though the Pandyan King possessed everything he was sad for he had no children and a rightful heir to the throne. King Malayathuvasa Pandyan on the advice of many Sages started performing many 'Yagas' and completed 99 'Ashvamega Yagas' the most holiest and difficult to perform of all the Yagas. Indra who knew that anyone who performed a hundred Ashvamega Yagas was fit to be the next Indra or Lord of the Angels, fearing that his post was becoming untenable, appeared before the King and advised him that performing the 'Puthrakameshti Yaga' was the most apt one and would immediately bear fruit.

The Pandyan King immediately after consulting Vedic-Pandits made necessary arrangements and after collecting the necessary articles needed started performing the Sacrifical-Fire ritual on an auspicious day and time. Even while performing the Yaga there appeared and sounded many auspicious sights and sounds that was a harbinger of good and noble tidings. The right-shoulder of the King started to twitch while the left-eye of the Queen similarly started to twitch and milk started to copiously flow out of her breasts (bringing about hormonal-changes in her body) and just then, out of the Yaga-Kunda (Sacrifical Fire-Pit) appeared a smiling, charming beautiful three year old girl.

The Divine child was dressed in a beautiful silk dress and pearls, rubies, sapphires, emeralds and diamond jewellery adorned her. She instantly stepped out of the fiery-pit, walked toward the queen and sat on her lap. The Queen, King and everyone assembled there were overjoyed and the queen hugged and kissed the child as if it were her own. The King then noticed that the girl had three breasts and instantly he was saddened for he in spite of giving away numerous alms and performing many pujas and worship and was treading that his foes would mock him for instead of a son who would claim his throne, here was a girl and that too an abnormal one with three breasts! Immediately there sounded an '*Asareeri*' or Divine-voice from the sky that claimed that he was to name the girl 'Thadagai', bring up the child just as he would with a boy-prince, train her in all the arts, archery, fencing, wrestling etcetera and when she grew up should make her sit on the throne as the reigning-queen. When the time was ripe, a suitable bridegroom would lay claim to her arm when her third breast too would disappear! He was not to feel sorry for everything was the Will of the Divine!

The joyous Pandyan King and Queen ordered no taxes were to be collected for seven years, all the outstanding and future taxes that were to be paid by the sub-kingdoms were also done away with and all prisoners were released as a good-will gesture. Alms and charities were given away manifold times and the entire city of Madurai and the entire kingdom wore a festive look.

Princess Thadagai was trained in all the sixty-four arts that included all sorts of warfare, literature, poetry, prose, music, dance, engineering, medicine…. And she excelled in them all! When she turned eighteen, she was crowned Queen of the Pandyan kingdom. She immediately mounted her chariot and along with the entire army went and conquered all the kingdoms of south and north India. She conquered all the countries of the world. She then went to 'Indralokha' or heaven and fought against the Devas and even Indra the Lord of the Angels ran away fearing for his life.

Queen Thadagai's attention then turned toward 'Kailash' the realm of the Primal Lord 'Siva'. All the *'Siva Ganas'* or Lord Siva's assistants were beaten and the Lord's chief aide 'Nandhi Deva' hastily approached the Lord to seek his protection. The Lord Himself came forward to battle Thadagai. Upon seeing the tiger-skin clad Lord with the 'third-eye' and the Crescent-Moon and Ganges adorning His matted fire-red locks, the third breast of Thadagai disappeared! She who had faced and fought the bravest and fiercest of warriors, stood with downcast-eyes with love and shyness overwhelming her! Thadagai's minister 'Sumathi' who was present when the Divine-Voice had claimed that her third breast would disappear when she met her bridegroom, without hesitation reminded her that He the Lord was the One she was going to marry! And instantly the Lord too claimed that she should go back to Madurai and he would come to claim her hand on the following monday!

The Lord as proclaimed arrived in Madurai with all the Angels and Lords of the 18 evolutionary cycles and the "seven upper and seven lower worlds" to claim her hand. And thus the Lord also known as 'Somasundarar' ruled over Madurai as 'Sundara Pandyan'. "What more needs to be said of the holiness of the Divine Temple of Madurai" claimed Thilagavathy for the Holy Father and Divine Mother themselves ruled over Madurai and its kingdom!

Appearance of the "Seven Seas" (Oceans) in Madurai; The dead King Malayathuvasa Pandyan brought back to earth from heaven in a Vimana; The King and Queen Kanchanamalai attain the Divine Form of the Lord and Divine Mother and leave for 'Kailash' the Ultimate Heaven

Heidi requested Thilagavathy to explain to them in brief about some of the 'Lilas' or Divine Sports that were extraordinary miracles enacted by the Lord in Madurai. Thilagavathy duly led them to the exact spot where the Lord ordered the waters of the seven seas (oceans) to assemble together to facilitate the Queen-Mother Kanchanamalai to bathe in them and thus purify herself.

Thilagavathy continued: "During the reign of the Lord as Sundara Pandyan and the Godess as Queen Thadagai, many Saints, Yogis and Sages came to Madurai to seek the blessings of the Lord and Godess. One among them was the Sage Gautama who as a show of respect paid a courtesy call to the Queen-Mother Kanchanamalai. Gautama was provided with a golden throne to sit on, provided with the necessary refreshments and the overjoyed Kanchanamalai fell at the feet of the holy Sage, paid obeisance and sought his blessings. The Queen-Mother further requested Gautama to explain on how was one (a sinner) to cross the deep ocean of sorrow being the earthly-life.

The Sage Gautama replied: *"You the devoted wife of the late King Malayathuvasa Pandyan have through your penance and Yogic-Powers attained the Divine Mother(who has given birth to all of nature) as your loving daughter and the All Pervading Lord Himself as your son-in-law!*

You being such a Yogi nothing would be unknown to you and You'd need no lessons on penance, Yoga, meditation and such, but since you asked me I'll tell You! Penance is of three kinds: 'Manadhal' - performing with the mind, 'Vasigam' – performing with words and 'Kayigam' – performing with the body. Thinking of performing giving away all sorts of alms and charities, compassion, patience, speaking the truth, silently meditating on Siva, controlling the five senses are performed by the help of the mind. Chanting the five-lettered Mantra of the Lord, uttering the Vedic-Mantras, singing in praise of the Lord, explaining about the great 'Dharmas' or eternal cosmic laws are performed with the help of words. Performing Siva-Pujas, Circumambulating clockwise the holy temples, maintaining and cleaning Siva-Temples, constructing temples, going on holy pilgrimages, performing holy cleansing baths in holy waters like the river Ganges and in oceans are performed with the help of the body. Among these three divine benefits, performance of bodily acts are of the highest order. And even among these bodily acts, bathing in holy rivers is of even a higher order. Taking purification baths in oceans where all the holy rivers merge is the ultimate!" Thus claimed the Sage Gautama.

The Queen-Mother kanchanamalai at once desired to bathe in ocean-waters so she called upon her daughter Thadagai and expressed her desire to her. Thadagai approached the Lord in guise as King Sundara Pandyan and not wishing to part with her mother explained her difficulty to the Lord. The Lord who had earlier during their marriage party brought forth the 'anna kullhi' (great mounds of curd-rice appear out of cracks in the earth) to satisfy the hunger of his humble servant 'Gundhotharan' who had earlier consumed all the immense quantities of food prepared for hundreds of thousands of guests and when whose thirst could not be quenched even after drinking all the waters of all the wells and lakes surrounding Madurai, had on His command made all of a sudden the river 'Vaigai' flow out of the exact spot where Gundotharan was ordered to place his hand whose roaring waters eventually quenched his thirst, instantly desiring to fulfill His wife's dear mother's wishes, the Lord thought of not one, but all the seven oceans to come in an instant and merge within a huge tract of land that was a dry lake.

Immediately with the deadly sounds of conches blowing and with foam and froth swirling seven huge fountains of water gushed out of the earth in seven different colors and sharks, dolphins and countless species of fish swam in its waters! The people of Madurai trembled with fear for they thought that it was the end days of the world for the roaring waters of the seven oceans rose in waves that were mountain-high and shook the very foundations of the earth! Immediately on the Lord's desire, the ocean waters calmed down and settled down peacefully as a placid lake.

The massive lake that contained within it the waters of the seven oceans was surrounded by a *"beautiful garden densely-filled with sweet smelling sandal, kumkum, manthira, mango, maghizha, pathiri and such plants and trees.* Scores of shrubs, creepers and plants filled with sweet-scented flowers rendered the very air with a pleasant odor. The Lord and the Queen were seated on a golden-throne among such pleasant surroundings and were being offered with freshly plucked flowers, drinks and snacks by a retinue of servants. The Lord addressed his dear Queen: *"My dear! As per your wish I've brought forth the waters of the seven oceans, please invite your mother to come over here and perform her cleansing bath!"*

The Queen-Mother Kanchanamalai instantly came along with the Queen filled with joy with the thought that her desire was going to be fulfilled and that too not just a cleansing bath in the waters of one ocean but in seven all brought forth due to the compassion of the Lord her son-in-law! She looked around the distinguished persons assembled there and asked the priests, scholars and Vedic-Pandits on what was the procedure for performing such a cleansing bath. The Pandits addressed her: *"Your majesty! The shastras say that one should enter the holy waters with one hand holding the son's hand, husband's hand or the tail of the holy cow!"*

Kanchanamalai was greatly saddened to hear the Pandits words and she with agony whispered in her daughter's ears: *"what a sinner Iam, my position is such that neither without a son or a husband, I have to grasp the tail of a female calf to take a cleansing bath!"* The Queen explained her mother's difficulty to the Lord. The Lord out of pity and compassion instantly thought of the late King Malayathuvasa Pandyan who was seated alongside Indra the Lord of the Devas or Angels in 'Devalokha' sharing the same throne.

Instantly a shining Vimana appeared on to which the Pandyan King stepped into and the ariel-craft flew down to earth and landed before the Lord! Upon sighting the Lord, the King ran towards Him to fall down at His feet and seek His blessings, but the Lord thought since he was His father-in-law and out of respect hugged him smilingly and pointed out his daughter the present Queen Thadagai and his beloved wife Kanchanamalai standing beside him.

The King hugged his daughter and said that though he was greatly saddened that he could not be there in person to see her getting married to the Lord Himself, he was now overjoyed to see them now as the Divine couple! His gaze then turned to his beloved wife Kanchanamalai who was dumbstruck with joy to see her late husband return back from the dead and that too from heaven!

Dressed as newly married couples and according to the Vedic guidelines, a smiling Kanchanamalai and the Pandyan King holding hands, entered the ocean-waters to take their cleansing-bath. Upon returning to the shore, they stood together and the Lord as Sundara Pandyan looked at them with compassion and Lo Behold! The couple turned into the exact replica of the Lord Siva and the Divine Mother Uma Maheshwari! As the Vedas claim that when one attains salvation and reaches the Lord's realm and/or His Presence, one attains all the qualities of the Lord and even 'Transfiguration' takes place, similarly everything turned out to be the Truth!

Similar to the Lord, the Pandyan King had 'three-eyes' (one in centre of the forehead known as the 'third-eye' *'Moondram kann'* and as the 'Forehead-eye' *'Netri Kann'* in Tamil), blue-hued throat (*'Neelakandan'*) marked by quaffing the poison that arose along with ambrosia when the "ocean of milk" (*'Parkadal'*) was churned, and with four-arms! A dazzling radiant golden-Vimana appeared from 'Kailash' the Primal heaven and holy realm of the Lord and the Pandyan King and Kanchanamalai boarded it. Like a young calf separated from its mother, the lucky couple looked with loving and longing eyes at the Lord and the Divine Mother even as the flying craft rose into the skies! The craft rose with cries of 'HARA HARA HARA!' rendering the air, conches sounding with all the Angels and heavenly hosts showering them with flowers and in a moment traversed 'Bhulokha' (the realm containing amongst others our solar system), then 'Bhuvarlokha',

'Suvarlokha' (1st heaven), 'Maharlokha', 'Thabalokha', 'Sathyalokha'(the Creator Lord Brahma's realm), 'Vaikuntalokha' the realm of the 'Sustainer' Lord Vishnu or Narayana and finally reached 'Kailash' the realm of the Primal Lord.

The Queen Thadagai thanked the Lord with her heart full of love for she had requested one ocean while the Lord had brought forth all the seven oceans; out of deep compassion had brought back her father from heaven; had provided liberation to her parents and moreover gave them the Lord's likeness (in figure and Qualities) (*'Siva Swarupa'*) and moreover ruled over the Pandyan Kingdom in Person, Madurai indeed was the most blessed place on earth and elsewhere!

Heidi and Shyam were also indeed blessed to stand on such sacred soil, they thanked their guide and philosopher Thilagavathy and looked in wonder at the very spot where the waters of the seven oceans appeared (which till three decades ago existed as a lake but has now turned out to be a big shopping-mall and only the street bears the name) and a temple known as the 'Kanchanamalai Temple' dedicated to the Queen-Mother which still stands in testimony to the great happenings that occurred in Madurai many millennia ago!

The Lord as a Siddhar who moved mountains, made an elephant statue come to life and consume sugarcane

During the reign of 'Abisheka Pandyan' the Lord with compassion and with the intention of providing the people of the Kingdom with both worldly and heavenly pleasures and blessings, appeared in the form of a Siddhar. He wore a tiger-skin as a robe and dressed Himself in saffron-colored loins worn by monks. His head was covered in knots of matted hair, holy-ash was smeared on the forehead, huge ear-rings, crystal-stone chains and the sacred-thread adorned him. A golden-colored staff in his hands made him look even more majestic and handsome to the bewitched people.

The Siddhar appeared in busy streets, street-corners, stages and were ever people gathered in large numbers across the streets of Madurai and began to playing mind-blowing tricks. He would be sighted in the southern part of the city and all of a sudden he'd disappear and appear in the north, he'd again appear in the east and all of a sudden appear in the west! Even as people in large numbers watched this spectacle in wonder, he would disappear for a longer period of time. He'd bring distant mountains closeby, make closeby mountains move far into the distance. He'd turn old people young and young people old! He'd convert men into women and women into men. He provided children to the infertile. The handicapped, blind, deaf, dumb and senile were all cured of their ailments. Through alchemy he converted base metal into gold. He made the riches of the rich and famous appear in the houses of the poor. He made friends without any reason fight among themselves. He made bitter-tasting fruit-bearing trees bring forth sweet and delicious fruits. Even though it was un-seasonal, he made the river Vaigai flow in spate and flood the dry plains and then made them dry again. He converted the sweet waters of ponds and lakes turn into salt-waters of the seas. The salt-waters

41

of the sea was converted by him into sweet waters. He flung his staff into the sky and stood with one big toe of his balancing on a needle stuck in the staff and performed many acrobatic-stunts balanced in such a way! He then placed his head on the needle and swirled furiously standing up side down! He flew into the skies, pulled down the clouds and wrung them as if they were pieces of wet cloth and squeezed out the moisture they carried! He made the moon and stars that appear at night to appear during the day. He would constrain the velocity of water, fire and air. He would bring forth buds, flowers and fruits that were all unseasonal in nature. He would by gently rubbing his staff on senile old men convert them into handsome young lads and also convert their aged partners into beautiful maiden and make them pregnant by offering them holy-ash! By sprinkling holy-ash on to the tounges of un-learnt people, he'd convert them into the masters of the "64 arts or branches of knowledge". He converted the coconut trees of the gardens of the King's palace into palmyra trees. And he converted animals, birds and trees one into another!

The people of Madurai were all bewitched by the antics and miracles played by the Siddhar and most of all were enchanted by his handsome features and the magnetic hypnotic sight of his eyes! People followed him in large groups ignoring their work and families. The King hearing about all this through his many spies, sent out his royal emissaries to welcome him to the palace and perform before him, but all proved in vain for the messengers themselves forgot their orders and followed the Siddhar! The King finally sent his most trusted ministers to welcome the Siddhar, but the Siddhar refused to accompany them and replied that *their King had nothing to offer or interest him!*" The ministers repeated exactly what the Siddhar had told them and the King too realized that Siddhars who had the blessings and grace of the Almighty would not respect even the devas and gods and hence would never ever show interest in him a mere king!

The Pandyan King realized his folly and chided himself to expect a 'Mahan' a truly great person and a full-blown Yogi to come and meet him in the palace instead of he going in person to meet him! The King out of great devotion and reverence left for the Madurai Meenakshi Sundareswar Temple and the Siddhar in an instant reading the King's mind and intentions immediately went to the holy Temple and sat on a spread-out tiger-skin in the north-west portion of the temple.

The King's guards and emissaries drew out their staffs and swords and ordered the Lord in Siddhar's guise to move on as the King deserved respect. As the Siddhar did not budge and sat on his tiger-skin with a look of boredom and what seemed to be arrogance and the King realized that this person was indeed a 'Siddhamoorthy' or a full-blown Yogi, a Perfected Being!

The King asked the Siddhar his name, his native place or town, what were the tricks and supernatural powers known to him and what was it that he wanted. To this the Siddhar replied: *"My dear fellow! I have no name and I'm not from any particular place! I roam around all countries and their towns. But still Kasi (Benares) is the town I dwell in now. Siva's devotees are my family. Day to day I roam around many villages and towns, display my magical-stunts and from Kasi I have moved southwards to worship at the Siva Temples. My dear fellow! This blessed place Madurai is the most sacred one on the entire earth and this holy Temple provides Wisdom to the true seeker. This un-comparable, purest and holiest of all holy Temples provides 'Jivanmukthi' (liberation even as one lives in the physical) and 'Paramukthi' (Divine Wisdom and thus 'Likeness' and 'Oneness' with the Lord) in the after-world. I'm performing my lilas (Divine sports) for the people this city and country and providing them with whatever they desire. I'm a master of the 64 arts or branches of knowledge and a full-blown Yogi, so I require nothing from you, Pandyan King!"* replied the Siddhar with a hint of a smile on his face.

The King's face turned red with anger and thought within that no one should be so arrogant with the belief that he knew everything! He desired to know the cause for such over-confidence on the part of the Siddhar. And at the right moment, a farmer ran to the King and offered him a long ripened sugarcane. The King immediately addressed the Siddhar and pointed out to a stone-statue of an elephant and challenged the Siddhar to make the stone-elephant consume the sugarcane. If he were able to achieve such a feat, he'd accept the Siddhar to be the greatest among all the Siddhars and even accept that he indeed was Lord Sundareswar, Lord Siva! Moreover he'd give the siddhar anything that he desired!

The Siddhar upon hearing the King's words and challenge thrown at him, smiled a little and replied to the King: *"Pandyan King! I desire nothing from You! I can provide you everything until all your desires are fulfilled! Persons who possess even one supernatural power, go to worlds where no one can, exhibit their powers and are honored by one and all. But I who possess all supernatural powers desire nothing. As desired by you, see for yourself this stone-elephant consume the sugarcane!"* Saying this the Siddhar glanced at the statue.

As soon as the Siddhar's sight fell on the statue, the stone-elephant turned alive! With sounds like thunder the elephant trumpeted, its eyeballs rolled over in all directions and with musth (hormonal-liquid) flowing out of its gland in its head, it reached out its trunk to the Pandyan King and plucked away the sugarcane held in his hand, stuffed it in its mouth. With juice and saliva over-flowing from its mouth the elephant chewed and swallowed the contents. The elephant then kept swinging its trunk hither and thither and swung side to side. The Siddhar's gaze once more fell on the elephant. The elephant instantly stretched its trunk to the King and plucked the pearl necklace adorning the King's neck! The King's angered guards raised their staff to hit the elephant and the Siddhar too glanced at the elephant in anger. But the elephant swallowed the pearl necklace!

The King was furious and greatly angered at the Siddhar and the elephant's action and his bodyguards raised their staff to hit the Siddhar. The Siddhar with a smile called out to them: *"Stop a little!"* The bodyguards froze as if they were statues and couldn't move their feet or a muscle! The King's anger vanished and his surprise and amazement grew manifold! He asked forgiveness of the Siddhar and saying this fell at his feet! The Lord who is an ocean of compassion and always melts when love and devotion is displayed and with deep compassion asked what was it that he desired. The King replied that he desired for a son who could justly rule the Pandyan Kingdom after him. The Lord blessed him with the words that it will be so, and placed his blessed hand on the elephant and gave it a look filled with compassion. The elephant brought forth the pearl-necklace that it had swallowed and offered it back to the King and immediately turned back into the stone-statue it had previously been!

Heidi and Shyam stroked the stone-elephant gently that Thilagavathy pointed out to them and tried to vision and enact the scene that had unfolded at that very spot thousands of years back!

Lord Siva made His Statue plant the left-leg to the ground and raise the alternate right-leg instead to fulfill his devotees wish

Thilagavathy asked Heidi and Shyam whether they wanted to see for themselves another rare sight and after getting their affirmation led them to the statue of Lord Siva performing the 'Cosmic' Dance.

In the Pandyan Kingdom lineage, Rajasekara Pandyan followed Vikrama pandyan. Rajasekara Pandyan was not only an excellent ruler but also a unique artist. He possessed great love and devotion towards the Lord and in particular loved the Cosmic-Dancer that was Lord Siva. His love and passion towards dance and particularly the Cosmic Dancer made him study and become master of 63 arts leaving aside one which was the art of dancing!

During the same age, the nearby 'Chola Kingdom' was ruled by the famous and versatile King 'Karikala Cholan' (who more than two thousand years ago built the famous 'Kallanai' dam built of stones and mud which still stands testimony to his engineering skills). King Karikalan was a master of all the 64 arts and his love of Lord Siva the Lord of dancers knew no bounds. During that time a poet of the Chola Kingdom who was on a pilgrimage visiting all the holy temples by foot, met the Pandyan King. He told the King that his King was a master of the 64 arts and unlike him was an expert in the art of dancing. The Pandyan King felt great sorrow and felt deep within his heart that Lord Siva wished him to learn and master the art of dancing also.

He went in search of great dance masters and after showering them with gold and other valuable goods began to learn dance. Even as he progressed in the art, he felt many a pain over various joints and parts of the body and particularly in the legs. The King then began to ponder, The Lord the

Cosmic Dancer who prevented and wiped away the birth pangs and many of life's pains of billions and billions of life-forms too must undergo pain of many sorts. Though it was not right to put an end to the Cosmic Dance of the Lord which in turn would mean the end of all the five acts of the Lord – the art of Creation, Sustenance, Destruction, the art to Veil and the art to Grace. Further the King felt that the Lord must feel discomfort and pain for he (as in all statues showing one raised leg) stands with the right-leg planted on the ground with the left-leg raised always.

As it were, that day happened to be 'Mahasivarathiri', the most important and auspicious day for Lord Siva's devotees. The King like everybody else fasted completely that day and visited the Lord's holy Temple that day and performed in all the four main Pujas spread over the day and kept awake in the night also. At mid-night, the Pandyan King rose both his hands above his head in prayer and with tears flowing down his face cried out to the Lord and prayed that to show compassion upon him and relieve the pain he must be surely undergoing, the Lord must plant instead his left-leg on to the ground and raise his right-leg or else he would throw himself on to the sharp-edge of his own sword which he had firmly stuck into the ground and kill himself. The Lord showing mercy on the King and out of deep compassion and love to his dear devotee instantly changed his leg-position and raised His right-leg instead! To this very day only in Madurai's holy Temple the Lord's statue stands with alternate legs raised to stand testimony to the fact that He bows to His devotee's wish and desire!

The Lord in Madurai gave 'Upadesa' (initiation) on the 'Ashtanga Siddhis' – The Eight Great Supernatural Powers to His Devotees

The Lord was seated in Mount Kailash (in the Himalayas on earth, 'Kailash' is also the Primal Heaven and holy realm of Lord Siva) eons ago (for this very holy mountain rose and rose repeatedly during and after each world-level destruction and deluge that burnt and then flooded everything on earth once every 'Kalpa' – the day-time of Lord Brahma the Creator which happens to be 4.32 billion years). The Lord was seated beneath a 'Kallalamaram' (a particular species of the banyan- tree) along with the Divine Mother, with the four Vedas (in living physical form), Bringu, Lord Nandhi Deva and other Sivagana Heads and the four "mind-born sons" of Lord Brahma – Sanaka, Santhana, Sananthana and Sanarkumara who were all seated obediently before Him.

All the Rishis were listening with fascination to the Lilas explained by the Lord Himself which all were as sweet as life-giving nectar. At that moment, the six 'Karthgai' Stars whose living-form were six bewitching women who had earlier fed their breast-milk to Lord Kartikeya or Muruga and also as Skanda the son of the Lord who in turn had been Created by six sparks that emanated out of the 'Third-eye' of the Lord. The six 'Yaksha' (one among the 18 evolutionary cycles) women bore the 'Rudraksha' beads and the holy-ash which are all the holy symbols of the Lord. They stood with humility before the Lord, bowed to Him and requested Him to give them Upadesa (initiate through silence and by either through 'mudras'which are certain particular finger or body symbols and/or movements or by uttering mantras or by mere power of sight alone where knowledge or wisdom is transferred instantaneously) to them on the 'Ashtanga Siddhis' – 'the eight great supernatural powers'.

The Lord in turn pointed kindly to the Divine Mother seated beside Him and said: *"She is the All Pervading 'Parashakti' the "First and Foremost Energy". Starting from 'Anima' all the eight great 'Siddhis' (Perfections) serve Her with humility. If you meditate on Her, She would absolve you of all your previous sins and provide the eight great siddhis!"* He then kindly gave them Upadesa (taught, revealed) of the eight great supernatural powers.

But as fate would have of it, the six divine-women forgot the knowledge or wisdom of the eight great supernatural powers revealed to them by the Lord! The furious Lord instantly cursed them with the words: *"All the six of you will turn into rocks and lie in the village of 'Pattamangai' under a great banyan tree!"* When with great sorrow they asked when they'd be absolved of their sin and overcome the curse the Lord replied again: *"After the passage of a thousand years I'd come to Madurai and absolve you all of the curse, let you regain your former physical selves and clearly initiate you on the Ashtanga Siddhis (eight great supernatural powers)!*

The Six divine-women as cursed by the Lord Himself instantly turned into six rocks below a great banyan tree in the village of Pattamangai. In due course of time fallen leaves, muck and dirt completely covered the six rocks. After a thousand years the Lord out of kindness and compassion appeared there in the form of a teacher of wisdom. He graced them with a kind look of compassion and immediately they (the rocks) regained their original-form! Their hearts were filled with love and joy as soon as the compassionate look of love the Lord fell on them. The six divine-women fell at the feet of the Lord to seek His forgiveness and the Lord too who is an ocean of love and kindness, touched them and placed His hands on the crown of the heads who earlier had nurtured Lord Kartikeya by letting him drink their breast-milk. The Lord then clearly initiated them and clearly explained to them the eight great supernatural powers.

The Lord gave His explanation: *"My children! Anima, Mahima, Laghima, Garima, Prapti, Prakamyam, Istvam, Vasitvam are the 'Ashtama Siddhis' or 'Ashtanga Siddhis – the eight great supernatural powers. The ability to turn one's body tinier than an atom that can dwell within the tiniest of life-forms is known as 'Anima'.*

The ability to permeate and expand into the 'tattvas' or principle-elements of the five 'boothas' or basic-elements in nature – earth, water, fire, air and space and also the 36 tattvas that make the physical as well as finer and spiritual bodies of man that also contain the '5 Siva tattvas' or the elements and qualities of the Primal Lord, is known as 'Mahima'.

The ability to weigh less than a feather that floats on air though the 'Siva Yogi' assumes the form of the incredibly heavy Mount Himalaya is known as 'Laghima'.

The ability to weigh as heavy as Mount Himalaya though the Yogi assumes the form of a 'paramanu' – smallest part of a split atom, is known as 'Garima'.

The ability to teleport instantly in a jiffy to any of the worlds and heavenly bodies of the "seven upper and seven lower worlds" and even beyond is known as 'Prapti'.

The ability to transmigrate into other bodies, travel and live in space; bring all that he desires where ever that might be, besides him; staying where ever he is and by the light radiated out of his own body, to know the 'three times' (past, present and future happenings) and know about all things on earth and in space is known as 'Prakyamaym'.

The ability to function like the Primal Lord by creating, sustaining and annihilating as and when he desires; by making the sun, nine planets; their satellites and all heavenly bodies to abide to his commands is known as 'Istvam'.

The ability to charm and bring under his control all life-forms that include plants, birds, animals, humans, life-forms of the '18 heavenly hosts' – the 18 evolutionary cycles is known as 'Vasitvam'.

My children! The Yogis who have realized Me will not desire to possess these eight great supernatural powers. Yet, these supernatural powers would follow them like shadows and exhibit their greatness to the world!"

Thus the eight great supernatural powers were very clearly revealed to the six divine-women. They in turn meditated upon the Divine-Mother as ordered by the Lord and thus were made capable to function if and when required with the Ashtanga Siddhis or eight great supernatural powers in their possession. The Yaksha women by getting the blessings of the Lord and the Divine Mother immediately attained both physical and Spiritual Liberation and hence having to go no more in the agony-filled endless cycle of death and birth, in a jiffy attained the realm of the Lord, 'Kailash'.

The World and its mountains excepting the Holy Temple and hills surrounding Madurai submerged by the rising tides

Thilagavathy went on to explain how very ancient Madurai and its holy Temple were to Heidi and Shyam: "After the reign of many Pandyan kings and the famous 'Suguna Pandyan' like all the just Kings before him too attained liberation and thus reached the abode of the Lord. After him twenty two Pandyan Kings reigned over Madurai. The twenty second King Adhula Keerthi's son was Keerthipudanan and it was during his reign the 'Maha pralaya' or great flood and catastrophic-destruction took place. All the seven mighty oceans of the world rose in fury in unison and their hissing black-waters completely inundated the entire world. The mighty eight elephants that guard the eight cardinal directions, the eight mighty mountains, the 'Sakravallha giri' (a mighty mountain), all the mighty nine-continents, the 'saptha' or seven Islands (continents), all its life-forms, all things material, all the high hills and mountains were destroyed. Excepting the 'Madurai Meenakshi Amman' holy Temple, the 'Indra Vimanam', the 'Golden-Lotus Pond', the 'Rishaba Mountain'(formed by the 'Lila' or Divine Sport of the Lord), the 'Elephant Hill'(which still exits), 'Naga Hill', 'Pasu Malai' and 'Pandri Malai' escaped the deadly onslaught.

After the great deluge and the flood-waters had drained away, the Lord Parameshwaran once more wished to Create everything "*as it was previously.*" He Created the 'Vinnavargal' the beings of space the 'Devas' or Angels and all others of the "eighteen evolutionary cycles", birds, animals and man. He once more Created the Kings of the Chera, Chola and Pandyan Kingdom. Among them the Pandyan King 'Vangiyasekara Pandyan' arose in likeness of the 'Full-Moon'.

King Vangiyasekaran built a small beautiful city surrounding his ancestors holy temple of Sundareswarar or Lord Siva. He ruled over the highly protected city in accordance to the rules framed by 'Manu' the ancient and great social reformer. During his excellent reign without internal or external enemies the country flourished in various ways. The flourishing people and their newer and wonderful constructions could no more be contained within the constraints of the small city. As wealth multiplied manifold, the population too exploded and his people needed more space to live comfortably.

The King went to the holy temple and standing before the Lord, prayed: *"My Lord by your grace and compassion my people and the Kingdom are flourishing but there remains one wish to be fulfilled. All the people need more space to live comfortably in. Like the ancient city ruled by my forefathers, I wish to build a larger city. Myself nor my ministers nor anybody else know the boundaries that previously existed. My Lord I pray to you to clearly mark the boundaries for the extended city!"*

The Lord who is omnipresent, but simple and is the personification of Love and Compassion, immediately appeared before the Pandyan King in the form of a 'Siddhapurushar' – a full-blown Yogi. The Lord who bore serpents all over His body, addressed the deadly poisonous snake that adorned His hands as a wrist-band: *"You shall go forth and measure and mark the boundaries of this great city as it existed previously!"* The snake in turn replied: *"My Lord by your grace, You should allow this holy-city to be addressed by my name!"* The Lord who is an ocean of Love said: *"It shall be so!"* The snake immediately went in at first eastward, after extending its tail to a great extent, after exactly reaching each and every boundary, it folded its tail and grasped it by its mouth to facilitate the marking of the four boundaries by the King's servants. After marking of the boundaries had been completed, the serpent once more adorned the Lord's hands and the Lord as a Siddhar went back to the holy Temple and disappeared into the Holy Figure of the Lord!

The Pandyan King at once began the task of constructing sky-high walls surrounding the huge city as marked by the serpent adorning the Lord's hands. The boundary to the south of the city was the present-day town of 'Thiruparankundram'; the 'Rishabakundram' hill marked the northern boundary; 'Thiruvedagam' marked the western boundary and the present-day town of 'Thiruphuvanam' marked the eastern boundary. The extended boundary-wall was known as *'Allhava madhil'* or 'Snake-wall'. And the city too became to be known as *'Allhavai* 'or 'Snake-city' or 'Serpent-city'.

The Pandyan King constructed once more huge walls to mark and protect the holy Temple; huge towers and beautiful ponds also adorned the temple's immediate vicinity. The King also made beautiful crowns and other jewel-studded gold ornaments to adorn the Lord and he reveled when performing such holy-tasks. Various people from all over the world came traded and lived in Madurai thus making it prosper to equal and then even transcend that of 'Alagapuri' the capital city of 'Kubera' the Lord of riches and 'Amaravathy' the capital city of 'Indra' the Lord of the Devas or Angels."

So you cannot even imagine how ancient and blessed is this city of 'Alavai'or Madurai, for it had even existed before and after the world was destroyed and created yet again after the great flood, said Thilagavathy proudly!.

Dharumi a Poet is awarded a thousand gold-coins; Nakeerar the Court-Poet is burnt by sparks emitted out of the Lord's Third-Eye; Narkeerar regains his normal previous self near the 'Golden-Lotus Pond'

Thilagavathy then led the couple to the 'Porthamarai Kulam' or the 'Golden-Lotus Pond' where millennia ago Narkkerar the court-poet regained his normal previous self and went on to narrate in brief about the famous sport played by the Lord, Dharumi the poor poet and Narkeerar.

The Pandyan King Vangiyasoodamani came to be known as 'Shenbaga Pandyan' for he had planted an entire garden full of 'Shenbaga' trees whose sweet-smelling flowers was utilized as the most preferred one for performing Pujas for the Lord in the holy temple of Madurai. Though the King had a vast collection of various varieties of sweet-smelling flowers that bloomed in plants, creepers, bushes, trees and in water-borne plants that were spread across ponds and lakes in his various large gardens, the preferred choice was the shenbaga flowers.

There were public and private gardens and the citizens of Madurai and its Kingdom often thronged the beautiful gardens to get away from the heat of summer and further swim and laze about in the scores of fountains, ponds, pools and lakes. The King and Queen too often found solace in their private gardens and on one such mid-summer day the royal-couple were in their private garden 'Chandrakantha'- a particular type of cool stone-house that was surrounded by many lilly and lotus-filled ponds. The couple were happily resting in each other's company at dusk when the moon was gently rising in the skies and the cool westerly-winds pregnant with the sweet-smelling odor of a very rare perfume floating past them gently soothing them to a light-sleep.

The King was gently aroused by the rare sweet odor which he had never ever experienced before. Even as the King was pondering over the rare odor, he was perplexed and felt that the odor was of divine-origin. He looked around and as he saw the Queen's spread-out hair, he noticed that the sweet-odor indeed originated from the Queen's hair! He also wondered whether the sweet-smell was caused by the usage of scented-oils and other such unnatural sources or were they the natural-odor of the Queen's hair!

The King later announced before the 'Tamil Sangam' in the royal-court and its many poets, musicians and seers that any person who could poem a song explaining on the source of the sweet-odor (that even the honey-seeking bees and beetles wouldn't be aware of) he had experienced in the palace-gardens, would be awarded a thousand golden coins! And duly a thousand golden coins was hung from the 'Porkillhi' or 'golden-parrot', being the symbol of wisdom, to be rightly claimed.

'Dharumi' was an orphan and a poor poet who was a devotee of the Lord. Dharumi prayed before the Lord and requested Him to provide him with a song that would enlighten the King on to the origin of the strange-odor experienced in the royal-garden so that he could claim the prize of a thousand gold coins. The Lord out of kindness and compassion appeared before Dharumi as a Siddhar and gave him a song written on a palm-leaf.

The song of Dharumi was read out in the royal-court which was greatly appreciated by one and all and the King too was completely satisfied by the song which ran like this: *"You beetle who possess beautiful wings and whose sole purpose in your entire life is to hunt and realize various odors! State the truth without fear nor favor, does any of the multitudes of odors experienced by you be comparable to the sweet-odor borne by the hair of the Pandyan-Queen who resembles a beautiful peacock and bears lovely chiseled-teeth?"*

Just as the thousand gold-coins suspended as the 'Porkillhi' in the hall of the 'Tamil Sangam' was about to be claimed by Dharumi, Narkeerar the

Court-Poet stopped the act and claimed that the poem was a flawed-one! When everyone including Dharumi questioned him, Narkeerar claimed that the words and grammar were correct but the contents were wrong. Dharumi ran to the holy Temple and standing before the Lord prayed with sorrow that a poet like him had found fault in the Lord's poem and for the good of Tamil and its future the Lord should confront the Court-Poet and debate about the contents and rectify the injustice caused! The Lord immediately appeared as a rich Poet adorned in fine robes and priceless jewels.

The Lord and the Narkkerar confronted each other in the halls of the Tamil Sangam. When Narkeerar claimed that no woman on earth or in heaven could have naturally sweet-smelling hair, the Lord asked whether that could be true for all the ladies and goddesses of the fourteen worlds, Narkeerar counter-claimed that it would be the same even for the hair of the Holy Divine Mother who always was beside the Lord to whom he daily prayed! When the Lord opened a little of His Third-Eye present at the centre of His fore-head in anger, Narkeerar claimed that even if he like 'Devandran' the lord of the Angels had eyes all over his body or even if He were the Primal Lord Himself and even if He completely opened His Third-Eye and burnt him to ashes, the fault in His poem was there for everyone to see! The Lord out of fury opened His Thirrd-Eye completely and Narkeerar was thrown to the banks of the 'Golden-Lotus Pond' with deadly burns all over his body!

The Pandyan King Shenbaga Pandyan along with other poets like 'Kapilan', 'Panan' and others in large numbers went in search of the Lord who had disappeared inside the holy Temple. After everyone cried out and prayed to the Lord who was the most loving and compassionate One, the Lord appeared along with the Divine Mother and claimed that He had come only to Play with Narkeerar in Tamil and restored him to his previous self. Narkeerar requested the King to present Dharumi with the thousand gold-coins and the King willingly gave him the award with much more in abundance!

Agasthya along with his wife 'Lobamudrai' flies to Madurai from the 'Pothigai' Mountain on his Vimana and teaches Tamil grammar to the Pandyan Kingdom's Royal Court-Poet 'Narkeerar' on the Lord's Advice

Narkeerar by the Grace of the Lord once more served with humility as the Chief Royal-Court Poet in the Pandyan Kingdom in Madurai. Narkeerar was thankful to the Lord for forgiving him and he thought that earlier when 'Manmathan' (Cupid) the Lord of Love was similarly burnt to ashes by the Lord, neither Lord Brahma the Creator nor Lord Vishnu the Sustainer had come to his rescue, but it was beside the 'Porthamarai' or 'Golden-Lotus Pond that the Lord Himself had forgiven him and restored him to his previous self. So from that day on Narkeerar took three cleansing baths in the holy pond and then went into the holy temple to pray to the Lord. He greatly repented for daring to challenge the Lord and thus earned the Love and compassion of the Lord.

Even as the Lord in Kailash His holy realm was pondering on how he was going to teach good Tamil and its grammar to Narkeerar, the Divine Mother reminded the Lord that earlier when the balance of the world had been disturbed (when the axis of the world had shifted and the south had risen and the north had sunk), He had asked 'Agasthya' the Sage *whom He considered to be equal to Himself* to go in the southern-direction to set right the balance. She again reminded the Lord that it was to Agasthya that He had earlier taught Tamil. When He ordered Agasthya to go south, he had told you that the people of the south spoke the Tamil language and were most proficient in grammar and prose and so he should also be taught proper grammatical-Tamil to converse with them and you out of compassion had did so, so he was the most suitable and able person for the job.

The Divine Mother also explained that Agasthya had earlier asked Him when was he again going to get 'Padha Dharisanam' (blessings of the Holy Feet of the Lord) with the Lord and He had asked Agasthya to pray towards Him in the 'Kadamba vanam' (the 'Kadamba tree-filled forest' that existed prior to Madurai being built there), get His blessings and all that he desired and proceed to the 'Pothigai Hill' along with his wife Lobamudrai. Agasthya was ever present there in the Pothigai Hill along with his beloved wife Lobamudrai, reminded the Divine Mother and if it was His desire, he could ask Agasthya to come to Madurai and teach proper Tamil to Narkeerar.

The Lord was most pleased by the Divine Mother's words and thanked Her for reminding Him of events and happenings that had taken place a long time back. Even as the Lord thought with kindness and compassion about Agasthya, the holy Seer along with his beloved wife Lobamudrai, *"got on to his 'thavam' (Penance) which was his vimana and flew through space"*, got out of the flying-craft and presented himself before the Lord within no-time!

Narkeerar after taking his thrice a day cleansing bath in the 'Golden-Lotus Pond' arrived in the holy temple to seek the blessings of the Lord and was taken by surprise and overjoyed to see the Lord along with the Divine Mother and the Sage Agasthya waiting for him! The Lord requested Agasthya to teach clearly proper Tamil grammar to Narkeerar which the great Sage did most proficiently. The Lord was very pleased with Agasthya and so patted him on the back out of kindness, presented him with many boons and left for His realm and Agasthya along with his beloved wife Lobamudrai once more left for the Pothigai Hill.

In Kailash, the Divine Mother asked the Lord why He himself had not taught Tamil to Narkeerar and asked Agasthya to do so instead. The Lord replied that one should teach to persons who worshipped Him every day, to those who gave away alms out of generosity, those who were not jealous in nature, those who kept their word and those who possessed a clear and faultless mind. Since Narkeerar was jealous, He had asked Agasthya to teach him Tamil! The Divine Mother felt happy after having her doubts cleared and Narkeerar too felt happy that even though he had envied Dharumi the poor-poet and dared to defy the Lord Himself, the Lord out of compassion had forgiven him and asked the great Sage Agasthya to teach him Tamil grammar! Narkeerar thereafter corrected his previous mistakes and remained ever faithful to the Lord and served with humility in the Tamil Sangam in Madurai.

Foxes were converted into Horses and Horses again into Foxes to show to the world the Faith of Saint Manickavasagar

After the reign of scores of Pandyan Kings, during the reign of Arimarthana Pandyan, in Vadhavoor a beautiful town on the banks of the sacred river Vaigai was born Thiruvadhavoorar later to be known as Manickavasagar. The town of Vadhavoor itself was a rich and fertile place and apart from its richness caused by the plentiful-crop borne regularly by its rich soil, it was always filled with the constant sounds and smell of countless Pujas, Yaagas and many Sacrifical-rites going on.Thiruvadhavoorar himself was born in idyllic-conditions in a priestly-family and by the time he was sixteen years old, he had mastered the *Vedas* and "*the 64 'Arts' or branches of knowledge.*"

Having heard of the talents of Thiruvadhavoorar, the Pandyan King invited him to his palace, presented him with many valuable prices and made him a minister in his court. Since Thiruvadhavoorar knew not only the 'Manu Shastras', he was also proficient in the books of weapons and warfare and so became an ideal choice to become the Chief Minister. Moreover many near and far Kings to befriend and get acquainted to Thiruvadhavoorar, became an ally of the Pandyan Kingdom and presented many priceless and rare gifts to the King.

Thiruvadhavoorar though holding very high, powerful and prestigious positions and did not lack in riches, was never entrapped in those luxurious and heady situations. He began to realize that even reading the Scriptures and Vedas and even holy books and texts of other religions were never going to help him overcome ego and get out of the endless cycle of birth and death. As the Vedas themselves say, not seeking material-comforts and the contented-life whether here nor in heaven, one should seek only 'mukti' or liberation, and to seek it earning the compassion of the Lord through devotion was the only way and means.

While the Chief Minister was yearning after the Truth and reading many Scriptures and meeting many learned people of Wisdom who happened to visit Madurai, with the thought of the Lord always in his mind, he attended faithfully to his court duties also. As the time for his Calling neared, in accordance to the Lord's plan, the Pandyan army needed hundreds of fresh imported breed of horses as many had grown old and inter-breeding had weakened them greatly. The King ordered his Chief Minister Thiruvadavoorar to draw as much gold and other valuables as required from the royal treasury and go to the harbors and purchase as many quality horses as required. He did so accordingly and before packing off many camel-loads of gold and other priceless gems, went and took a cleansing bath in the Golden-Lotus Pond and prayed at the Lord' holy temple to help him utilize the royal-funds to help him subdue his senses and for the welfare of the Lord and His devotees!

As Thiruvadadavoorar neared 'Thiruperunthurai' his heart began to melt and a strange joy filled him. The Lord appeared as a Guru seated under a 'Kurundhai' tree along with many devotees. Thiruvadavoorar forgot everything else and joined his master and started spending all the money meant for purchasing horses, to repair the Siva Temple and perform many Pujas, Yaagas and many other forms of worship. The Lord pleased with the 'gem-like' words chanted by Thiruvadavoorar, named him as 'Manivasagar' and/or as 'Manickavasagar' – "the chanter of pearl-like words".

As days went by and the money started to drain away, the worried Manickavasagar went into the temple and prayed to the Lord as to what he was to do as the Pandyan King was expecting the fine breed of horses. The Lord replied as an 'Asireeri' or a "voice from the sky" stating that he should order his royal-servants to go back and tell the King that the horses would be coming shortly. After ordering all the soldiers and palace-workers who had accompanied him to return back to Madurai and tell the King that the horses would come shortly as stated by the Lord, Manickavasagar went on performing Pujas and worship.

After the passage of a month's time, the King sent a messenger to enquire when the horses would be coming. Manickavasagar after getting a reply from the Lord went in person to Madurai. After taking a cleansing bath in the Golden-Lotus Pond and praying to the Lord, Manickavasagar went to the palace to meet the King. Pleased to see his Chief Minister after many months, the King asked how much gold and valuables he had taken with him and how many fine horses he had purchased for them. Manickavasagar replied: *"the amount of gold taken was infinite and the number of horses that would come would also be infinite and they would like the Sun-god's seven-horses be victorious-horses!"*

The King was extremely happy and presented his minister with many valuable gifts and eagerly anticipated the arrival of the horses. But the family of the minister chided him and asked him what was he going to do tomorrow when the horses were not delivered, Thiruvadavoorar the minister now known by the name Manickavasagar replied in the way a person who had renounced everything in the world. He said that after the Lord had out of compassion and grace had appeared before him in physical-form though He was formless, he had renounced everyone close and dear to him. Renounced pain and pleasure. Renounced the body and its cravings. Shunned all things material. Shunned off anger and ego.Renounced the fruits (merits and de-merits) gained by performing good and bad deeds. He had realized that father, mother, teacher were all but the Lord. All living-beings are his family and the Lord's devotees are his close-ones and taking birth again is to be hated and shunned the most. He said that he had the utmost faith in the Lord, entire humanity was his family, Entire Mother-earth was his bed. A simple loin-cloth was his attire, Holy-Ash alone was his balm for the body and the 'Rudraksha' (bead-garland) was what would adorned him. Death would be welcomed at any moment. The King can punish me or exalt me, pleasure-filled heaven or pain-filled hell would make no difference to him. He would never forget the Lord who had showered him with love, grace and compassion. Who could prevent him from experiencing the fruits earned by committing good or bad deeds in previous moments (and births)?

Manickavasagar who had renounced all those near and dear to him, had let go of his ego and was constantly in communion with the Lord was invited to the palace by the King and questioned on when he was going to deliver the horses. He replied that the horses would arrive in three days and that the King should order the construction of huge stables to house the tens of hundreds of horses with many tanks, ponds and deep canals to be dug to facilitate the horses to quench their thirst and be exercised. Everything was prepared as ordered by the King within the stipulated time of three days and moreover the entire city of Madurai was festooned and decorated and lamps were lit allover to welcome the horses.

When the horses did not arrive after three days the King became furious and cursed himself for not heeding to the warnings of his spies and ministers when they had stated that there never were even signs of the horse-transactions and that his Chief Minister had spent all the money in other endeavors! The King ordered his guards to imprison the thief that surely was his Chief Minister and torture him till he returned all the money, gold and other valuables he had withdrawn from the treasury. The guards and soldiers of the pandyan Kingdom made Manickavasagar bear huge boulders of rock oh his head, but since he bore the Holy Feet of the Lord, the weight of the boulders did not affect him in the least. The torturers wondered at this marvel and pondered whether they were witnessing something magical and supernatural! At night Manickavasagar's hands and legs were cuffed and was whipped for hours on end, but nothing hurt him as held strongly to the Lord's feet (which according to the Yogic-texts exists above the crown of man's head).

As dawn broke, the sound of ringing bells and Siva-mantras being chanted in the holy temple was heard distinctly within the prison chambers. Manickavasagar called out to the Lord in pain and asked him when he was going to be delivered from the wretched conditions in jail and give him liberation. The Lord too out of compassion felt that the time had neared for His devotee Manickavasagar's deliverance and immediately ordered the Chief of the 'Siva Ganas' that were always besides Him to take along the leaders of the Siva ganas and go inperson to the forests around Madurai, turn all the foxes there into horses and proceed towards Madurai. The Lord said that He too would accompany them as the prime trader of the horses.

As willed by the Lord, all the foxes of the wild were turned into fine thoroughbred Arabian and other region's horses and all the Siva ganas rode them wearing fine attire. The Lord Himself rode the finest of the horses attired in white linen, a royal turban and wore priceless jewelry all over His body. The horses were so majestic and bewitching to look at that all those who saw them with captivating eyes felt that the Kings of the bordering countries of the Cheras and Cholas and their generals and captains would all envy them. Even their King's heart would burn for daring to suspect and torture his own Chief Minister who had made such a fine purchase! All the charming ladies who happened to see the Lord immediately fell in love with the charming bewitching handsome figure and lost their hearts to Him! The dust rose like a great cloud when they were about five miles or so from Madurai and a few soldiers guarding the fort-ramparts of the city rode ahead to inform Manickavasagar and the King about the impending arrival of the horses!

The guards accompanied Manickavasagar to meet the King who was in the happiest of moods and with a huge smile hugged his minister and presented him with a priceless pearl necklace. The King sat on a golden throne on top of the ramparts of his fort-walls under shade and was eagerly anticipating the arrival of the war-horses. In accordance to the Lord's Will and as time went by and there were no sign of the horses, the King sensed that he was like numerous times before being fooled by his Minister and with fury rising manifold as time went by, made a sign to his guards who immediately dragged away Manickavasagar and began to torture him again!

Manickavasagar cried out to the Lord again and prayed that people would mock at the Lord who did not come to his devotee's defence! Even as he was being tortured, hordes of the 'Maya'(illusive) horses arrived raising a cloud of dust. The Pandyan King was stunned at seeing those magnificient creatures and once more received his Minister with joy and claimed that there could never be another person more loyal and trustworthy in performing his duties and spoke to him in endearing tones! The Lord in the guise of the chief trader rode a magnificent horse that was none other than the Vedas taken to life as the creature and claimed to the King to see Him ride the horse in the most skillfull manner. He rode the horse in five varieties of steps and eighteen wonderful types of prances and trots.

The awestruck King enquired as to who was the chief trader and the Lord full of radiance rode before the King. As soon as the compassionate and grace-full look of the Lord fell on the King, the King's mind went blank for a moment, forgetting who he was, he rose from his throne and raised both his hands above his head in prayer and total surrender! After a moment remembering who he was, he felt ashamed that he had rose and paid respects to a mere horse-trader and not knowing what to do stood near his throne. The Lord then claimed: *"My dear King! Your Chief Minister Manickavasagar who always keeps his word, gave to me and for my horses piles and piles of gold and for that I've brought herewith high-breed horses of excellent qualities bought in various countries in faraway places! Please listen to the general rules that are utilized in horse-trade. After receiving the reins from me as of today, they become yours, I take no responsibility on the condition of the horses hereafter. There would be no court that could settle any arbitrary cases that you would bring on me in regard to the trade that has been settled today. This is the custom generally agreed upon in the horse-trade."*

The Pandyan King agreed upon those terms after inspecting and seeing for himself the fine condition of the high-breed horses. The Lord explained the various high qualities of the different breed of horses and ordered his 'Siva ganas' to ride their horses in front of the King to admire and appreciate the beauty of the horses trotting past him. The King was immensely pleased to see the skill and agility of the horses. The Lord then advised the King that the horse-exchange ceremony should be conducted after performing pujas. The King had all the horses decorated and smeared with sweet-smelling sandal-paste, decorated with garlands of flowers, adorned them with quality saddles, stirrups and reins. Incense-sticks and camphor were lit and after vermillon was smeared on the forehead of the horses, pujas were conducted and the smiling Pandyan King was prepared to receive the horses from the Lord. The Lord after raising both His hands and praying in the direction of His temple, handed over the reins of His horses one by one to the King. After receiving all the horses excepting the Lord's own horse that was none other than the Vedas in living-form, the King ordered all the horses to be rubbed-down, fed and housed in the newly built royal-stables.

The King threw a white cloak in the direction of the Lord who having decided to save His devotee got down from His horse, picked up the cloak and tied it as a turban to adorn His head. The King accordingly presented all the horse-riders with costly attire and after receiving them, the Lord who rode the magical-horse and His loyal servants disappeared. The King also presented his Chief Minister with many prizes as a mark of respect and returned to the palace.

Manickavasagar returned to his house with musicians and a band leading the way and young women dressed in finery with lit lamps accompanying him. After all friends and relatives had left him, Manickavasagar went back to meditate on the Lord. He was greatly pleased and satisfied that the Lord out of love and compassion had come and saved him and brought forth fine horses to justify his spending of the money and gold of the royal-treasury in the upkeep of the Lord's House. His only other desire was for the Lord to help him remain always in service of the Lord and forever in his mind.

As night came, due to the 'Lila' – divine-sport or game of the Lord, all the beautiful horses regained their previous form! They (the foxes) felt sorry for being imprisoned in the stables.They thought: *"We were reduced to the sorry-state of bearing heavy men on our backs! We had been chained and tied down by chains and ropes and received whip-lashes too! Did such a condition fall on us when we lived in the forests? When will we again hear the sweet-sounds of conches blowing, beats of the 'parai' – drums used in funeral-processions and the wail of women? There are no snails nor crabs here to satiate our hunger! We can no more eat grass, oats, pulses and grains! It would be for the best if we were to run away from this place before dawn!"* Thinking likewise all the foxes got loose of their ropes and chains and attempted to escape. They bit and tore away chunks of flesh of the old horses stabled there. When the stable-keepers opened the doors to see what was going on there as they heard the deafening howls of the foxes, all the foxes ran away!

Madurai city which was always known for and reverberated with the sweet-sounds of cymbals and bands, the sounds of elephants trumpeting in joy, the sounds of horses trotting past, sounds of mantras chanted in sweet-Tamil and the songs of 'Panars'(Divine song practitioners), was instead filled with deafening sounds of foxes howling in the still air! All the gardens, orchards, streets, temples and mansions and palaces were filled with foxes in large numbers! Some foxes entered the kitchens of houses, scattered about utensils and vessels and ate the food remaining there. Some bit and ate alive the chickens, pigeons, parrots, sheep and pig reared by the people. When dawn broke and the gates of the fort-walls surrounding the city were opened, all the foxes ran away into the forests!

The next morning the prison guards, the palace guards and the King's personal body guards including all the ministers were all terrified as to how they were going to inform the courage to explain to the king about the night's happenings. But still they mustered courage and went up to the King and with quivering voices spoke: *"Your highness! The wonderful horses that rode like the wind which arrived yesterday all turned into foxes in the dead of night. They escaped prison after tearing the living flesh of all our previous horses, ran into the city, killed countless hen, fowl, pigeons, parrots, sheep, pigs, cattle and caused havoc everywhere! They howled, bit everyone on sight causing panic and then vanished into the surrounding forests!"*

The enraged King screamed at his ministers and claimed that his own Chief Minister had deceived him by looting the riches of his treasury and by some magical means had turned all the foxes of the forests into horses and cheated him! He further asked his ministers on the type and quantum of punishment that should surely be awarded to Manickavasagar. The ministers all looked down in shame and couldn't reply to the King for the same punishment could turn towards them in a moment for previously praising the very same person! Just at that precise moment, Manickavasagar walked in with all thoughts centered on the Lord!

The King in rage spat out at his minister and asked how being born in a priestly family could he have committed such a dastardly crime. When Manickavasagar asked what had happened, the King repeated all that his guards and ministers had told him. He then ordered his soldiers to drag the disgraced minister to jail and torture him till he had returned all the money and gold he had looted from the royal treasury! The soldiers after tying Manickavasagar's hands and legs, made him stand face-up in the hot burning sunshine and made him bear huge rock-boulders on his face, forehead and chest. Manickavasagar bore everything and kept on repeating the Lord's Holy names even as the torture continued. The constant prayers and cries of His devotee made the Lord decide to act and show to the world His devotee's faith and by causing the Vaigai river to burst, flood her banks and the city and eventually cause a poor old lady named 'Vanthi' to attain both physical and spiritual liberation and fly before everyone's eyes in a heavenly Vimana to Kailash the Ultimate Heaven!

The Lord called upon the river Vaigai which was none other than another name and form of the river Ganges to burst forth like it would at the end days of the world and flood everything within Madurai. Vaigai immediately burst its banks and caused deadly destruction everywhere. All the soldiers and guards ran helter skelter to save their lives and their dear one's lives. Manickavasagar was left alone and he calmly walked in the direction of the Lord's Holy Temple, entered it and sat down silently unperturbed and meditating in peace and happiness on the Lord!

The Lord who out of compassion worked as a laborer to get 'whipped' by the Pandyan King and thus causing the pain to be reflected on all life-forms of all the worlds and thus explaining His Omnipresent-state and to liberate 'Vanthi' a poor old lady

The flood-waters of the Vaigai river rose dangerously high and as time went by the water level kept on rising. The people of Madurai were terrified as life-stock and property were all swept away in the rising racing waters. King Arimarthana Pandyan called an emergency-meeting of his ministers and top officials to take stock of the alarming situation. Soldiers and the public were ordered to heighten the banks on either side of the river. Trees were cut down and were laid down parallel to the fast flowing river-waters. Bushes, leafy-branches of trees and hay were packed tightly in the gap between the trees and sand thrown in to somehow bolster the temporary dams being hastily built on the river-banks to try and stem the flow of the rapidly rising waters. But all efforts failed and the people watched as the flood-waters rushed at a even more rapid pace into the city!

More and more people were ordered to roll hay and stuff them in the gaps and loads of river-sand was dumped in to try and raise the river-banks. The 'Parai' drums were sounded and 'Victory Battle-songs' were sung to bolster the waning courage of the workers and the people. They cried out to the 'Mother' (most river-gods were considered to be feminine-gods) river Vaigai as to what caused her to become so furious and angry enough for her to vent her fury against the people and live-stock living along her banks!

In the south-eastern part of Madurai lived a poor old lady named 'Vanthi' who was in her eighties. She had no relatives of her own, but possessed great love and devotion on the Lord. She was of a loving-nature and was like a mother to all. She made tasty 'Puttu' (sweet rice-cakes) every day and only after with great love and devotion offering and serving the delicacy to the Lord, would go into the streets of the city to sell them and earn a living. Vanthi's poor but contented simple-life was suddenly disturbed by the sudden floods of the Vaigai river. The King's soldiers had sounded the Parai-drums and called out to the citizens of Madurai to appoint at least one person per family to help stem the floods.

Vanthi who had neither family members nor friends to stand in place of her prayed to the Lord who was her last refuge as defying the King's orders would be tantamount to being declared an enemy of the state! The Lord who consumed the 'Avi'('Havis' in Sanskrit) - the food offered into the Sacrifical-Fires by Sages and Yogis and the food offered to Him personally by the Divine Mother, out of compassion rushed to His devotee's rescue like a hungry calf running to drink its mother's milk! The Lord wearing a dirty torn old piece of cloth around His waist, bearing a hay-strung ring (to evenly distribute the weight) on the crown of His head on which was placed an inverted bamboo basket and a mud-shovel hooked on to His shoulders appeared as a laborer in the streets of Madurai! He called out to see if anyone would hire Him to perform menial jobs and arrived in the street where Vanthi lived.

Vanthi came out of her house and asked whether He could dam the portion of the Vaigai river-bank which was marked-out as her portion. The Lord who had neither father or mother and came as a single person asked: *"Mother! I'd do the job, but what and how much would your quantum of payment be?"* Vanthi replied that she would serve Him 'Puttu', which she made and sold every day. The Lord in turn replied: *"Mother! Due to biting hunger I'm extremely tired, if you were to serve Me the unformed puttu (the powdered-remains left after the cakes were tightly formed by pressing them within one's fists) I'd eat them, take a bit of rest and perform my duty in double-quick time!"* Vanthi brought forth the unformed puttu, gave it to Him and in a kind voice asked Him to eat it. *The Lord began consuming the puttu and claimed: "Wow! What taste! What taste! It tastes heavenly and is even better than Mother's (breast) milk! This is truly the food of the gods and it*

is fit to be served to Lord Sundareswar (Lord Siva) of 'Alavai' (Madurai)"
The Lord even while shaking His head with nods of appreciation, ate the
delicious puttu laced along with her kindness and love!

The Lord claimed: *"Mother! You have done away with my hunger and
tiredness by serving Me with food laced with kindness, compassion and
the love of a Mother, whereas I Myself do not have a father or mother and
am all alone. I will bring you happiness and joy by immediately setting
forth to complete the job allotted to you."* And saying these words the Lord
proceeded towards the banks of the river Vaigai. He requested the officials
there to register His name as Vanthi's accomplice. The Lord by thought, by
word and by written-confession identified Himself (who is the Omniscient,
Omnipresent, Almight One) as a simple laborer!

The Lord then proceeded to shovel sand on to His basket, raise it to His
head and immediately dump it on the ground claiming that the load was too
heavy! The Lord would then shovel lesser amount of sand into His basket,
pretend to stumble and let the load uselessly fall down! He would then dump
a few head-loads of sand on the embankment, feel tired and sit down. The
heavy load would cause pain in His head. Blisters would form on His hands
they would turn red. Blood would seep from His holy feet. He would then
walk towards the shade of a tree standing on the banks of the river, place
the basket as a pillow, lie down and go to sleep happily!

The Lord in the guise of a laborer would then get up, start to sing in a
beautiful baritone voice! He would heap sand, dance on it and draw the
attention of all others in the vicinity. He would all of a sudden laugh away
merrily like a mad-man, suddenly sit down in a quiet manner. He'd run fast
in the sandy-banks letting the sand fly past Him. He would then drop to the
ground as if He were dead-tired, sweat heavily, inhale deeply and would
return back to Vanthi's hut hungry as ever!

To Vanthi the Lord claimed: *"Mother! The river-bank portion allotted to
you is being rapidly built! My hunger is still to be satiated, please serve
me puttu mother!"* Vanthi at once served piping hot puttu cooked just then
and the Lord downed the hot puttu that caused steam to emanate from his
bowels and mouth. Tying the remaining food in a knotted corner of His

towel, the Lord once more proceeded to the river-bank. He dug the sand with supposedly renewed vigor, but went and dumped them into other people's allotted portions! He beat his chest and shoulders in a show of triumph when He saw the dam-breaches holding fort against the flow of the current. He hugged persons close-by with joy! Once again he carried a basket-full of sand, tripped purposefully and fell into the rushing torrents. He swam back to shore after retrieving the basket and banged it against the banks repeatedly to dry it. He unwound the reeds of the basket and began to tightly wind them back again. The next time He would let the basket fall into the rushing torrents, leap into the water to retrieve it, get caught in swirling waters, grasp a floating log and climb back to the shores way down the river!

The Lord in the guise of a laborer would then lean heavily on his mud-shovel and inhale air in deeply as if dead tired. He would then unwind His towel, peer at the puttu, sniff it to see if it was okay and then start to consume it with glee! He would then offer the puttu to persons working close-by thus causing the work to be hindered. When the King's guards came with raised staff to beat Him, He would laugh and clap His hands in joy! The Lord who existed in the sky, in space, in sand, in women, in children, within all objects and who was seen by the *'Jnana-kann'* – "the eyes of Wisdom" of Yogis who themselves were desireless, had transcended their body and senses and realized the 'Absolute-Truth', was also seen in the Physical by the people of Madurai while playing His 'Lilas' – 'Divine Sports'!

At that time the Chief guards of the King arrived to inspect the ongoing repairs being done to the river-banks. They were comparing their notes with the designated names and their allotted portion of work. The banks were all raised sky-high with sand and packing-materials excepting the portion allotted to Vanthi. When they called out in anger to Vanthi, the Lord appeared before them handsome as a *'Ghandarva'* – a god! When water started to flow in through the gap and breach the remaining wall also they shouted in anger as to the reason why he had not completed His work, the Lord stood silent. When the rushing torrents started to demolish all the repair work done, they still hesitated to hit the stately figure! They wondered if *"He was a mad-man?" "Was He a possessed person?" "Had He come to cheat Vanthi?" "Was He a Siddhar (Perfected Being) performing 'Indra*

Jalam' (magic of the gods)?" "We cannot understand who He is?" "As a talented musician is He a Ghandarvan – a god?" "Is He a master of dance?" After not getting answers and their doubts grew manifold, they decided to report the matter to the King!

Even as they decided to proceed and meet the King, Arimarthana Pandyan the King arrived on the spot and they reported on the recent happenings! The King who was happy and satisfied to see for himself that the mounds of sand and packing had withheld the flood-waters turned furious upon seeing Vanthi's portion left open. The rushing torrents swept away all the good work that had been done! When the King enquired about it, the frightened guards got hold of the hands of the Lord and dragged Him before the King stating that He was Vanthi's representative.

The guards claimed that this handsome person had Himself claimed to be Vanthi's servant, registered Himself to be her accomplice and got paid in advance for the work to be completed. The King saw the tall stately figure who was even more handsome than 'Manmathan' (Cupid the Lord of Love) and though poorly dressed, looked like never having done any hard-work in the past! When the Lord did not answer to any of the questions put forth by the King, he snatched the gold-inlaid cane from the palace guard and whacked it solidly on the back of the Lord who is the universe and the Infinite containing all the worlds and all life-forms! The Lord in an instant dumped the sand along with the basket at the point of breach and vanished! The breached-portion too in an instant was restored successfully for the sand-mound rose to a dizzying-height!

The scar and pain caused by the Pandyan King hitting the Lord on His back was instantly reflected and experienced by the King and by his wife the Queen. It was experienced by the ministers, soldiers and guards. The elephants, horses, the sun, the moon, the planets, the stars, the five basic elements in nature, the clouds, the Vedas, the trees and forests and the Seers. The welt caused upon the Lord who exists as the 'Life' of all beings appeared on the Devas (Angels), Man, Nagas (beings of the nether-world), birds, animals, serpents, ants, hills, trees, creepers, grass and shrubs. Even the foetus were affected and after being born bore the welt. Even lifeless paintings bore the mark of the welt!

When the King's guards and soldiers arrived at Vanthi's house to arrest and torture her for sending a servant who performed incredible magical-feats, she prayed to the Lord to save her for she feared being tortured by the palace-guards in her old age. The most kind and compassionate Lord who had been lovingly fed by Vanthi, due to His grace, sent a wonderful radiant 'Vimana' (aeriel-craft) along with His 'Siva-ganas' (the Lord's accomplices). The craft landed and the Siva-ganas welcomed her with the words: *"Mother please come with us!"* With the sounds of five types of trumpets blowing, chants of sweet Vedic-mantras and Angels showering flowers on her, Vanthi boarded the craft and flew to Primal-Heaven 'Kailash' the Holy Realm of Lord Siva!

When Heidi asked Thilagavathy what then happened to the Pandyan King Arimarthanan and Manickavasagar, she continued her trilogy which included Shyam also. When the welt and pain caused by the King whacking the Lord on His back was experienced by everyone including the ministers and guards surrounding the King, they all displayed their injured-backs to him making everyone to wonder at their simultaneous punishment! The King too was perplexed and stood confused and at the same time afraid and terrified by seeing the great mound of sand that had appeared where the Lord had dumped His basket load of sand and disappeared in an instant!

His fear and worry turned to joy when the Lord through a 'Asireeri' – voice in space, spoke: *"My dear Pandyan! As all your money and treasures were earned through 'Dharmic' (Righteous) means and was pure in nature, it was given to Me and my devotees with great love and devotion by My blemishless devotee Manickavasagar! But you punished him. That is why I brought forth the foxes that roam the forests as horses. They once again ran away again into the forests as foxes at midnight. You again punished and tortured Manickavasagar. Unable to bear it I caused the Vaigai river to flood and breach her banks. I appeared as a laborer and as salary received the puttu given by Vanthi and got hit by you. After dumping one basket-full of sand and raising the banks and then disappearing, I removed the sorrow of Vanthi who is the personification of the love of a mother by giving her liberation and thus sent her to My Holy Realm! All these were done by Me for and on behalf of Manickavasagar! Little did you realize the greatness of Manickavasagar. He who has great devotion towards Me has provided to you an exalted life here on earth and in (Primal) Heaven! Let this exalted Pure person (Manickavasagar) act according to his wishes and you continue to rule this holy land for a long time!*

Thilagavathy went on to add that the Lord out of His kindness, love and Grace, subtly hinted to the King that he too like Vanthi was liberated from the endless cycle of birth and death! So, one should always remember to earn wealth through righteous-means and lead a selfless-life not expecting rewards for the services done to others (that includes services done to all life-forms)!

The Pandyan King then went in search of his minister Manickavasagar who was later found in the holy temple meditating on the Lord. The King fell at the Saint's feet and asked his forgiveness. The Saint in turn replied that there was nothing to forgive for it was due to the King that he was able to receive the love and grace of the Lord. He then proceeded to 'Chidambaram' to pray and meditate on the Lord and later compose 'Thiruvasagam'. Thiruvasagam greatly moved Rev.G.U.Pope more than thousand five hundred years later for him to claim: *"If Thiruvasagam did not melt one's heart, nothing else would ever will!"*

A Red-legged Crane (*Senkaal Narai*) attains Liberation, 'Transfiguration' takes place and thus attains 'Swayarupa', the Form of the Lord "with Four arms and Shoulders and Three-Eyes" and flies to Ultimate Heaven in a radiant Vimana a Flying Craft

Shyam and Heidi asked Thilagavathy whether the Lord gave Liberation only to humans or other life-forms as well, and she replied that though man was the most qualified being (with a fully-developed mind) the Lord had Liberated hosts of life-forms like a 'Karu Kuruvi'(a small black-bird native of southern India) and a Crane, apart from life-forms of other 'evolutionary cycles'.And she began to narrate the story of a crane which got deliverance from the endless suffering of birth and death.

In the southern part of the Pandyan Kingdom there was a prosperous and beautiful city filled with large domed multi-story buildings. In that city there was a large lotus-filled deep lake. The lake's banks were surrounded by large stone steps that led from the top right to its bottom to facilitate bathers to enter and exit the waters easily. There were a lot of fish in that lake and a 'Senkaal Narai' – a 'Red-legged Crane' caught and ate those fish and lived on trees bordering the lake's banks.

Once after several years of seasonal-rain had failed, the lake turned absolutely dry. The Crane which subsisted on fish alone, rose into the skies and flew at a rapid pace to search for water-filled bodies that would contain fish. After flying for a very long time, it fell down from the sky due to hunger and exhaustion in a dense forest. In that dense forest lived a noble-hearted blemishless Yogi and Saint known as 'Sathyatha'. He who was always in 'Siva-Consciousness' had attained a pure state of mind that was blemishless. Due to the grace of the Lord the Saint was always in a state of ecstasy. A group of 'Jivan Muktas' (Ones liberated even while living in their physical bodies here on earth) were always present with the Saint.

The forest contained a very large lake that was square in shape and had stone steps leading down to the bottom surrounding the lake on all four sides. The banks were lined with large shade-giving trees like the 'Shenbaga', 'Pathiri', 'Vengai', 'Vanji', 'Maghilam', 'Kura', 'Mara', 'Mullh Murungai' and 'Marudham' that all apart from giving dense cool-shade also emitted sweet-smells that arose from their innumerable flowers. The lake was known as 'Acchotheertham' and the Crane found refuge in the leafy-branches of the huge trees that provided a canopy all around the lake.

Even as the Crane was keenly observing the hordes of fish in the lake-waters jumping and frolicking about, a group of Hermit-Saints arrived to take their regular bath. The Crane was surprised to see that whenever the Saints rose out of the water after taking a dip the fish of the lake jumped and rolled playfully over their shoulders and in between their massive spread of hair in the water! The Crane thought: "*Ha! These fish would have to be really blessed and committed numerous good deeds and penances for them to even touch and be in close contact with such great holy-bodies! I should not hunt and consume these fish!*" Disregarding its hunger-pangs the Crane remained there.

The Saints after completing their bathing and other religious-rituals returned back to their huts. They went into the prayer-hall and started reciting from the holy-text that contained the stories of the 'Lilas' – the Divine-Sports enacted by the Lord Himself who as the first King 'Sundra Pandyan'and His lineage of Kings had and were enacting the holy deeds. The Saints beautifully sang the Praises of the Lilas played by the Lord, His Praises, His Infinite Love, Kindness, Grace and ease of approach shown towards His devotees who surrendered to Him whole-heartedly. They also sang on the uniqueness and greatness of the Holy Divine Temple of Madurai and the holiness of the 'Golden Lotus-Pond'. Upon hearing this, the Crane's ignorance lifted away like a curtain that had been drawn aside. Body, sense and mind-cravings were burnt away. Life-strengthening Wisdom blossomed. Its Love towards the Holy-Feet of the Lord grew to such an extent that it immediately took to flight towards the incomparable Madurai and reached it.

Remembering the sanctity of the 'Porthamarai Kulam', the 'Golden-Lotus Pond', it took a purifying-bath in it and went into the Holy Sundareswar Temple of the Lord. It circumambulated the Lord who stood under the 'Indra Vimana' (stone replica of the Ariel-Craft of Lord Indra the Lord of the Angels), stood before the Holy presence of the Lord and remained meditating on the Lord firmly entrenched within its heart. The Crane followed this ritual with utmost faith for fifteen consecutive days without consuming food (fish) or water. When it went to take its purifying bath on the sixteenth day in the Golden-Lotus Pond, it stood by its banks watching hordes of fish beautifully swimming, jumping and flying through the air and falling back again into the clear waters with a flash.

The starving worn-down Crane thought of catching and consuming the easy succulent prey, and in a flash due to the Infinite Grace of the Lord, like a spark intelligence dawned in it. It thought with deep sorrow: *"Oh God! How could I even think of consuming the holy fish living in this holy and incomparable lake? When will this birth come to an end?"* It went into the Holy Temple and even as it began to meditate on the Holy-Feet of the Lord, the Lord who is beyond the reach and understanding of the greatest of the Devas (Angels & Gods) appeared in the very Form that the Crane meditated upon! The Lord asked: *"My devoted fellow! What boon do you desire? Put forth your desire!"* The blessed Crane bowing with Love before the Lord replied: *"My Lord! Please liberate me from this life of suffering and raise me to (the exalted-state) Your Holy Realm of 'Sivaloka' (Kailash) where Your true devotees are! Another boon I desire My Lord! Birds of my species as well as other ones of the future would be greatly tainted by the sin acquired by consuming the fish of this exalted holy-lake, so I pray to You that by Your Grace, no more fish should live in these holy-waters!"*

The Lord out of kindness and love toward His devotee granted the two boons prayed for by the Crane! Immediately a radiant Vimana (Ariel Craft) flew down from the Holy Realm of the Lord. The Crane was in an instant transformed into the *'Siva Swarupam'* - 'likeness' of the Lord with *"four-shoulders"* and *"three-eyes"* and with beautiful sounds of five-types of musical-instruments emanating and with the Devas raining down showers of flowers, the Crane rose into the heavens and in an instant reached the Holy Realm of the Lord to be welcomed into the exalted company of 'Nandhi Deva' (the Lord of the Siva Ganas) and the Siva Ganas for eternity!

Thilagavathy went on explaining to Heidi and Shyam: *"From that day, not only fish, but even other water-borne creatures do not live in these holy-waters of the Golden-Lotus Pond. And as wished by the Crane, not only cranes but other bird-species and other life-forms that take purifying-baths in this exalted Pond, by the Grace of the Almighty God easily gain the Love and Grace of the Lord! The Pandyan Kingdom and its people were thus absolved of their sins and Dharma (righteousness) flourished. Due to the faith of the Crane, the people and the King Suguna Pandyan attained the exalted 'Siva-State'!"*

The Pothigai Mountain

After profusely thanking their guide Thilagavathy who refused to take their monetary and physical gifts and explained that it was an honor and a passion to explain and elaborate on the Holy divine Sports of the Lord, Heidi and Shyam left for Mukkudal a hundred and sixty kilometers south of Madurai and twenty-five kilometers west of Tirunelveli town, being the home-town of the latter on their way to Pothigai Mountain.

The couple after being pampered for two days with home-made food and delicacies served lovingly by Shyam's parents left for Papanasam. On their way lay the town of Ambasamudram and the reason they stopped over there for therein was a very rare holy temple dedicated to the holy Siddhar Agasthya. They were fortunate enough to gain entry into the temple for it is shut down at noon and reopens only at four in the evening. After praying before the statues of the venerated sage Agasthya and his Russian-born (as mentioned by His Holiness the late Sankaracharya of Kanchi: *"the name 'Russia' was derived from 'Rishi' or the land of 'Rishis' – Holy Sages")'* Lobamudhra', the priest showed them a sealed-off room in which during the festival-time (held once a year) a huge mound of rice was placed and the room was padlocked for the night, only to find footprints of the Sage on the rice in the following morning and most of the rice being consumed!

Papanasam was a small town located at the base of the group of mountains known generally as the 'Pothigai Mountains'. As its name suggests Papanasam means "the place which destroys sins" ('Papa' – sins; 'nasam' – obliterates). And to wash away their sins and even more to cool off after their forty-five minute drive they both took a refreshing dip in the refreshingly cool holy-waters of the gently flowing river Tamiraparani. They then entered the Holy Siva temple that stood on the river banks for eons to pray to the

Lord and bless them with the sight of the holy Siddhar Agasthya who habited the blessed hills.

Even as Heidi walked over the huge steps that led into the temple admiring the more than thirty feet tall wooden doors that had beautiful carvings on it, Shyam pulled her back. Shyam pointed out to Heidi a large black granite stone that were plastered on to the stone walls on either side of the entrance. There on the stone were mentioned in Tamil and English that in the year 1938 Shyam's great-grandfather had donated Indian rupees five hundred for electrification and Rs.Two hundred for lighting the Holy temple. Shyam explained to Heidi that the sum of Rs.Seven hundred was indeed a great amount during those days during the British rule when a gram of gold cost Rs. One while the current price was more or less Rs. three thousand!

As they drove up the hills after signing in at the check-post of the Forest department of the 'Kalakad Mundanthurai Tiger Sanctuary', Heidi happily pointed out herds of spotted-deer known as chital to Shyam that were merrily grazing on the luscious grass that bordered the winding roads. They were even fortunate to have a glimpse of a group of red wild dogs chasing a Sambhar (moose like huge brown-colored deer) stag before vanishing into the thick vegetation. After driving up a couple of kilometers they reached a sharp bend and later could view the famous 'Agasthya waterfalls' that lay far below on the opposite side of a valley. Heidi enquired about the lady Saint who lived somewhere above the waterfalls that her dad had often mentioned to her about and Shyam pointed out to the trail of white-washed stone steps that was visible to them even from that distance. Shyam told her that he had heard that the Saint had habited a small cave, lived for more than 110 years and had attained the state of Samadhi a couple of years earlier.

Heidi reflected on her dad telling her about his meeting the Saint and on how she placed her hands on the rock-walls that surrounded the large pool that lay down and beyond the cave and repeatedly 'materialized' sweets and other snacks that was more than enough to satisfy the hunger of himself and the three other Europeans who had accompanied him.

By noon they had reached the 'Forest Camp Office' in Mundanthurai which also housed a British-style guest-house built along the banks of the river that flowed down from the newly constructed dam at Servalar a few kilometers upstream. Shaym and Heidi went and met the 'Forest Ranger' who welcomed them warmly for he had prior intimation from the D.F.O. (District Forest Officer) in Tirunelveli that the couple had got special permission to hike up to the summit of the Pothigai Mountain from the Chief Conservator of Forest himself! The Ranger glanced only briefly at the sanction order for he himself had one emailed to him a couple of days earlier. He also welcomed Mr.Purushothaman a sixty-five year old gentleman who had hiked up the hills and beyond for more than forty years and his dad 'Sundaram Pillai' like himself had been a guide and an ardent devotee of Agasthya for more than thirty-five years earlier!

The Ranger told the couple that Purushothaman was the most ideal guide for them for he knew the forest like the back of his hand and also knew the 'Kani' or the forest-dwelling tribal people personally, spoke their language and could get their assistance if and when needed. Purushothaman had earlier shown them photographs of his dad showing off his tiger trophy and told them that his dad had been the chief accountant in the Triuvanthapuram Palace in the nearby state of Kerala in the early 1900's and was lent by His Majesty the King of Travancore to the Zamindar of Singampatti (that lay a few kilometers to the east) to set right the accounts upon his humble request.

After having a simple but tasty and healthy vegetarian lunch at the forest guest-house the expedition left for the Karayar dam lying several kilometers up that was constructed by the British government and opened in 1938. The dam was somewhat circular in nature and several kilometers long and wide and its depth was 142 feet at its deepest point. The dam-waters had large quantities of fish as well as a few hundred crocodiles which were all let in by the wildlife-department. Most of the crocodiles that were let in when they were just babies were preyed upon by wild-dogs when they lay basking in the sunlit shores but the ones that had escaped were huge in size after several years of plentiful fish-feeding.

Heidi and Shyam stretched out their legs when they reached the dam and after sending back their car to Mukkudal took along their backpacks and along with Purushothaman and a forest-guard they left by motor-boat to traverse the length of the dam. Though there were several score of motor as well as row-boats lying on the banks, theirs was the only one that was allowed special permission to ply the waters. Purushothaman explained to them that a legal problem between the Forest department and the P.W.D or Public Works Department *and* the Fisheries Department had entwined all of them in legal cases in the Courts of Law and hence for several years the boats were not allowed to ferry passengers.

As it was the month of June, the south-west monsoon season had set in and therefore there was a slight drizzle of cool rain accompanied with welcome gusts of the famous *'thendral'* or gentle southern-wind. The boat-man warned Shyam to pull back his legs which he let them trail down at the cool water's-edge sitting at the bow as a crocodile might just take a fancy at his leg being a fish! Though they saw what seemed to be huge logs lying in distance, some were to their horror huge crocs that sank slowly into the water-depths as they approached. Purushothaman told them that there were never any incidents of crocs attacking humans for as long as he remembered and he too like many kids in the past had bathed in these very waters and he still did, but there could always be a first one and it was better to be careful when approaching any wild animal.

They reached the other sandy-banks after fifteen minutes or so and viwed the beautiful 'Vanatheertham' waterfalls whose waters that flew down from a heavenly pool of water lying more than fifteen kilometers upstream and right at the base of the Pothigai Mountain known as 'Poonkulam' being the Source of the Tambiraparani river. Purushthoman led them up a rocky trail to a safe place that had iron-railings to guard the bathers from slipping down the rocky-slopes to a deep pond where many careless bathers had slipped down, bashed their heads and died. After soaking in the cold-waters for a couple of minutes, they climbed still further up moist slippery steps and after several hundred or so feet reached a small cave naturally formed in the rocks and their guide Purushothaman claimed to them that this was the 'Judge Swamy Guhai' or (cave of the Judge) known to but very few persons!

The 'Tantra Yogi' who teleported to England and was back in a jiffy

On their way back to the boat and on their ride to a bamboo-grove that lay a few kilometers to the east, Purushothaman told them of the true incident behind the cave they had just seen. Sir John Woodroffe was a Judge during the British rule in India and was in Calcutta during the early 1900's. A Yogi was caught hold by the local people as he was found loitering in graveyards during night-times and was produced before the Judge. When the Judge questioned on what grounds the Yogi was arrested and produced before him, it was stated that he was suspected of practicing witch-craft and human-sacrifices! When questioned by the Judge in person whether the claim was true, the Yogi replied that among the various forms of worship practiced all over the world he practiced 'Tantra Yoga' that had nothing to do with witch-craft or human-sacrifice.

Sir John Woodroffe had read and heard of Tantra Yoga and knew that it produced potent power to the practitioner in a very short time. He asked the Yogi who looked very calm and composed whether he had attained 'Siddhis' (Perfections) and thus Supernatural Powers. When the Yogi replied in the affirmative, the Judge asked whether he could demonstrate some powers that he had attained. The Yogi replied that he could do so and asked the Judge himself to state on what Supernatural power was he to demonstrate. The Judge said that since he had heard nothing from his wife and children back in a remote part of England for more than six months and further had heard that a great fire accident had destroyed his entire village and its people, could the Yogi enlighten him of the safety and if possible whereabouts of his family. The Yogi replied that it was possible and that do so he should be provided with a quiet room and no one should disturb him for an hour or so.

All arrangements were made as requested by the Yogi and he went into the room and locked himself within. Upon returning after some time, he handed over a letter written by the Judge's wife claiming that the Indian Yogi sent by him met her and that only she and the children had escaped the deadly fire-accident while the entire village and its people perished in it! The astonished Judge Sir John Woodroffe immediately resigned his job and became the Yogi's pupil. He later meditated for twelve years in the cave at the Pothigai Mountain and later on wrote many books on Yoga, one being 'The Serpent Fire' and, 'The Garland of Flowers' another being 'The Maha Maya'.

Heidi and Shyam listened with fascination and wonder to the story narrated by Purushothaman as the boat gently touched the shores near the bamboo grove that was to be their immediate destination. They got off the boat and after sending back the boat who was heavily rewarded, they started to climb up and though the bamboo forest and after a few minutes reached a small trail that led to the 'Kannikatti Forest rest-house' that lay about seven kilometers further up. Though the trail they now tread on actually led from the Karayar dam that they had left an hour or so earlier right up to the Forest guest-house, their guide deliberately chose the boat-ride for the trail was a tiresome travel of twenty two kilometers of rocky bouncy jeep riding. Moreover Purushothaman wanted the couple to experience the boat-ride as well as visit the waterfalls as well as see in person the secret cave nestled in the hills.

As the group walked leisurely through dense cool foliage many exotic insects, birds, reptiles and animals revealed themselves. At first they could hear the chatter of monkeys and lion-tailed macaques revebrate across the hills.Many large 'Malabar red squirrels' skirted above them devouring fruits and spitting out the peelings, their reddish-tan skins and large fluffy tails glistening in the rays of sunshine that managed to penetrate the leafy-shade. Among the droves of pigeons and doves that they saw high up in the trees, Purushothaman particularly pointed out to them what seemed to be green-colored parrots when actually they were plump 'green- pigeons'. Only when the green pigeons moved among the dense leafy-branches could they be seen merrily tearing into luscious red juicy banyan fruits which were their favorite meal. Purushothaman told them that though these were small as parrots, there were huge ones that habited the denser regions of the forest which were as big as the kites and eagles that always dominated the skies of India hunting out dead rats and snakes.

Spiders and insects of various species, colors and sizes could be sighted and the forest-guard told them that there were poisonous bees, wasps, scorpions(particularly small white scorpions known in Tamil as 'Raja Thellh' or 'King scorpions'), spiders and beetles that caused instantaneous death. In fact a few decades earlier during the rainy-season in a village near Shyam's hometown, a large beetle struck a person on the forehead while he was partaking the wedding feast and instantly slumped down dead! Small green-colored snakes littered the forest-floor and they were so well camouflaged that they literally to avoid them at the last moment had to jump over them as they walked on. Leaches of various species and sizes latched on to any warm-blooded animal including humans and sucked-out blood in large quantities and they performed them so silently and painlessly that the victim never even noticed them and they dropped away only after gorging themselves with blood and becoming bloated like small suckling-piglets! Some leaches travelled through pants and trousers to the most impenetrable parts of the body and only by pouring salt on them or by burning could they be removed.

At one point there was some open space from where they could look down and across beautiful green valleys and lovely colorful hornbills could be seen majestically flying on as if in slow-motion. Larger animals could not yet be seen for it was still mid-day and even deer and larger game all rested in deep shade or in and near water-holes and streams. As they were about midway to their destination, they had to walk across a small culvert which was a stone-bridge built over a small stream besides which was a small clump of bamboo-trees. Purushotham cautioned to them to tread carefully and silently for a pair of King-Cobra snakes habited that grove and had many a time chased away persons during their mating and egg-incubating seasons. He further explained to them that King Cobras were the only species of snakes that built nests to facilitate incubation of their eggs. Even though no snake chased them they could hear the hiss of an angry snake which sounded more like an angry growl that warned them of the presence of the reptile, so they quietly but rapidly walked away!

After a couple of hours of easy walking they reached the Kannikatti forest guesthouse that was like ever since the British left, kept poorly maintained. Leaving their belongings at the forest bungalow and guarded by the forest-guard, Heidi, Shyam and Purushothaman walked down to a cold stream to take an invigorating bath. Purushothaman explained to them that his dad had showed him a place upstream where the British had diverted the stream-waters to flow directly underneath the bungalow to fill in their bathtubs and their cloak-rooms, but repeated floods had obliterated the temporary stone-dam.

It was turning dark rapidly as the sun set as it always does in Indian jungles so they rapidly walked back to the forest bungalow. The bungalow was built of stones and tile-roofing and had glass windows on all sides to light-up the place. The visitors had to do with battery and solar lamps for there was no electric supply available. While Heidi and Shyam had instant macroni with cheese for dinner, the two others who couldn't stomach such food had chappathis which were a sort of baked wheat bread along with pickles that they had brought along for cooking food in often wet rainy conditions was a cumbersome process.

At night though the bungalow had a small moat that was dug right around the entire perimeter of the bungalow to discourage any wild animals or snakes to cross-over, the two locals slept within the safety of locked doors while the two youngsters unrolled their sleeping-bags on the verandah and lay down to enjoy and experience the smells and sounds of the cool jungle atmosphere. As darkness enveloped them for additional safety they switched on a solar lamp to ward off any inquisitive creature, but in turn started to attract mosquitoes and moths and so had to quickly put them out! Late at night though they could hear the sound of barking-deer and the 'saw' of a leopard and even the throaty growl of a tiger hunting far in the distance they slept on till dawn broke.

As soon as there was adequate light to light their path and after brewing some coffee and drinking it hot while at the same time munching on some biscuits and dates, they quickly were on the road again. After walking for a couple of kilometers and crossing a few streams and an estate leased-out by the Forest Department that had plantations of cardamom and pepper, they came out across a huge open grassy field. Heidi and Shyam stood shocked, awestruck and astonished to see large herds of huge Indian bison known as 'gaur' grazing in the distance. The bison instantly became aware of their presence and though they looked up from their grazing for an instant, they soon lowered their massive heads to keep on munching on the rich grass. Though instinct warned them of close and present danger, as for the past couple of decades hunting had been strictly banned, the bison as well as other wild animals began to recognize humans as 'frendlies' and accepted them to be present at a safe distance. The visitors too realized their vulnerability and so avoided to never get within close proximity when bison, bears and particularly elephants could turn violent.

They set off again and soon ascended a gentle slope where they were bathed in cool breeze heavily scented with the odor of herbs and Shyam instantly remembered his uncle Sridhar telling him of the medicinal value of the air that was cool after passing over thousands of kilometers over the Arabian Sea and passing through innumerable herbs that these very hills were famous for. Shyam also reflected to Heidi on what his other uncle Suresh had told him regarding the sweetness and medicinal value of the Tambiraparani river waters, they were all mainly due to the herbs and particularly the countless number of gooseberry trees. It is said that the roots and bark of the gooseberry 'softens' the water that flows over it and to add to it copper was also present in the river-water which enhanced its taste and uniqueness. Ancient Indian texts also say that a very rare form of gooseberry fruit known as 'Karunelli' (literally 'black gooseberry') existed in these very hill which was the 'elexir' or the "fountain of youth" that was presented to the Saint-Poetess and Siddhar Auvviar by Emperor Adhihaman more than two thousand years ago.

The pathway that led to the base of the Pothigai mountain passed through groves of gooseberry and wild mango trees whose ripe luscious fruits were greatly sought after by not only birds and monkeys but by deer, wild boars and bear as well as elephants. In fact the group on purpose made loud noise and bantered so as to ward-off elephants and bears which were the most dangerous animals to be encountered by surprise out in the wild. Bears particularly suddenly without provocation would attack a person and rip off muscle and tissue and crunch on bones utilizing both its teeth and sharp claws. Elephants usually moved on but an encounter with a loner would usually end up with fatal consequences. As the group walked on wading across numerous streams and 'shola' forests that literally meant thick shady forests, the sounds of many small and large animals scampering away could be heard and only rarely could Heidi and Shyam point out particular animals for they were well camouflaged. Only once were they were able to spot a black bear moving in the distance and shortly a mouse-deer whose dainty-feet accomplished tremendous speed when cutting through thick undergrowth.

By ten in the morning they came across the famous and often quoted 'Sangumuthirai' ('Conch Symbol') symbolizing holiness carved into a large rock right at the base of the Pothigai Mountain. After taking a break for a couple of minutes they made the final dash for the mountain peak. The going was a bit tough for the rough steps if they were called to be that, were huge and it was more like climbing one rock on to another. After ascending a few hundred feet though the young couple felt nothing, Purushothaman who was in his mid-sixties was panting a little but the forest guard couldn't move a single step further for the constant pressure on the legs started to make them shake and tremble and so they left him there and started again imagining what the effect would be on the poor man when descending.

As they ascended further they stopped often to admire the beautiful scenery that unfolded before them. Opposite to their own peak, there was the equally imposing 'Naga Pothigai' (literally 'Snake or Serpent mountain') for the peak resembled the hood of a snake and 'Iynthalai Pothigai'('Five-headed mountain') stood majestically as if guarding the holy Pothigai mountain. From their vantage, Heidi pointed out six or seven large rocks on the slopes of the opposite mountain a few hundred meters away which suddenly moved and both Shyam and herself shouted out in unison 'elephants'!. The elephants couldn't hear them for the velocity of the wind carried off any noise and even then they were safe in the distance! The hills on all sides were covered in emerald-green forests and greenery which was truly a feast for the eyes.

The last hundred feet or so was really steep and an iron chain was suspended by some kind British climber of the past which greatly helped in overcoming the final few hundred feet or so. The peak itself was quite large and round in shape. Though it was rock, it had patches of grass and right on the peak stood a small statue of the exalted Siddhar Agasthya or Agasthiar as he is known in Tamil. The statue was open to the elements until a few years back but now had a roof over it. After Purushothaman had placed a few offerings of coconut and bananas and some sweets and garlanded the statute, the three of them prayed for the blessings of the exalted Sage.

Late in the afternoon after Purushothaman had left to pick up the Forest guard on his way down, Heidi and Shyam as per their wish stayed on at the peak for the night to if possible get the Grace and blessings of Agasthya in his physical presence. As they walked all around the peak and admired the emerald-green view that unfolded on all directions, they pointed out to each other interesting places they knew from their vantage point. Heidi pointed out the red-roof tiled bungalow that was the Kannikatti Forest bungalow that they had left a few hours earlier lying a little to the east of them a couple of thousand feet below them. Shyam quickly showed Heidi the two dams visible from there and a large pool of water lying right at what seemed to be their feet at the base of the Pothigai mountain on whose summit they now stood, which was 'Poonkulam' being the source of the Tambiraparani river. And what was even more interesting was since it was a cloudless-less clear day, they could clearly see the Arabian sea to the west while a hazy view of the Indian ocean to their south and the Bay of Bengal to their east was visible.

Later as they lay in the soft grass admiring the clear blue sky, sudden 'whup' like sounds that resembled rifle-shots brought both of them to their feet. Even as they were wondering on the source of the sounds emanating suddenly for Shyam was accustomed to the sound having seen 'tracer' bullets (to show the parabolic trajectory of the bullet's flight-path) being fired when his kid-sister Sabi underwent training in the N.C.C. (National Cadets Co.) and later in her rifle club and Heidi of course was not new to the sound as she had accompanied her dad when they went hunting for rabbits and deer back in Germany even when she was a kid. All of a sudden two small black figures shot past them flying high into the air and many others followed in quick succession. Both one after another cried out:'Swift'! Heidi had seen swift birds in the heights of the Alps as well as at 'Table Mountain' in South Africa when she had gone holidaying a couple of years earlier and Shyam had seen them at the 'White Cliffs' of Dover back in England. The swift was said to be the fastest bird in the world that could fly at 105 miles per hour in stable level flight but were capable of flying much faster when diving and were surprised that they existed in India. The birds rode the air with aplomb as they along with fine mist came down from the valley nearly kissing the rocky cliffs and rose hundreds of feet above the summit of the fountain flying vertically at tremendous speed that resembled the modern-day jet fighters as well as futuristic ones for their wings lay swept back and folded besides them like pointed scimitars, and after reaching their peak, once more fell back again to the depths of the valley to once again ascend into the skies!

Agasthya – 'Mushin' the state of 'no-mind'; Agasthya possessed and could enact the Five Powers of the Lord;

When it had turned dark both Heidi and Shyam after consuming only a few bananas and some water, sat bathed in moon-light and under a radiant star-spangled sky before the holy statue of Agasthya and meditated while keeping their attention focused at the tip of the nose and in alignment with their breath. Since both had attended 'Vipasana' classes run according to the 'Buddhist' tradition as well as by Zen Masters, they both quickly went into 'mushin' the state of 'no-mind'.

Although Heidi and Shyam had experienced the state of bliss while being in the state of no-mind, infinite bliss enveloped them and they were gently aroused into consciousness by an overwhelming sweet odor and gentle soft-music. As both of them simultaneously gently opened their eyes there sat before them the smiling radiant golden-form that was none other than Agasthya! Tears of joy overflowed from their eyes as they were in the presence of infinite Love, Light, Power and Compassion! They were in close presence of the Divine who possessed all the Five Acts of God: the Power to Create, Sustain, Annihilate, Veil and to Grace.

The energy emanating was to such a degree that both Heidi and Shyam were finding it difficult to breathe and they literally started to levitate for all normal laws of science like space, gravity, radiation, magnetism etcetera were negated in the holy Seer's presence. Only when the Sage smiled widely and asked them both to relax did they return back to their normal selves. It need not be said that a mere scowl or a frown countenanced on the Seer's face would send even planets and stars into oblivion and this was understood by both the visitors. The love and compassion emanated also would make dried and withered dead-crop as well as any life-form to spring back to life.

Only submission to the holy Sage with love and compassion filled in their hearts had helped the couple to draw in him, who was equated with the Primary Lord by the Lord Himself!

To make them at ease, Agasthya began to ask them about the well-being of their parents and friends though his deep but at the same time kind look seemed to suggest that he knew all the answers even before they were put forth. The Sage then asked them what was it that they desired. Although they should have asked for his grace and guidance to help them to be delivered out of the painful endless cycle of birth and death, they both replied that the holy Seer should clear many of their doubts. When the holy Sage smiled and nodded his head in affirmation, they began to question him.

Heidi: "Sir! Why this endless cycle of birth and death?" Agasthya: "This question has been in vogue for countless eons and not just of this world! All this is a 'Lila', a game a sport to the Lord! Although as quoted often in many ancient Indian texts as well as the Holy Bible, the eternal plan (of the Lord) is to convert the believer to attain the exact image (replica) of the Lord with all His qualities and return back to his true home which is Primal Heaven." Shyam: "Sir, You say exact image, have you not attained the image of the Lord and is the attainment of primal heaven an absolute necessity?" Agasthya: "The image is not important, only the *State* is, like Lord Krishna says in the Bhagavad Gita, He appears in the form desired and wished for by the devotee. And for the one who has attained the State, space and time becomes irrelevant, heaven is where he is!"

Heidi: "Sir! How many lives or should I say, how many births do we take, is it seven births?" Agasthya: "The Lord Himself in the 'Sri Shiva Rahasya' says that 84, 000 are the births and as pointed out by Saint Manickavasagar in his 'Thiruvasagam's' 'Siva Puranam', we take birth countless times passing through the lives from a blade of grass, shrubs, creepers, plants, trees, birds, reptiles, animals, man (as man itself he takes 6000 births) to a 'Yogi' or divine man, god (Angels), 'Maha Devas' or 'great gods' and finally the State of the Primary Lord Himself!"

Shyam: "Sir, why are there so many religions in the world? Are there many gods?" Agasthya: "The Lord is One while many are His aspects and Forms!

Not unlike the proverbial five blind men who all try to describe an elephant, each one describes the part he comes in contact with as truly the elephant, be it the ear, tail, trunk or leg! Only the person who has the power of sight (the realized or enlightened one) realizes that all of them are partially true while the Whole or Absolute Truth eludes them!"

Heidi: "Sir, is religion a must to attain the Absolute Truth? Agasthya: "Absolutely not! What is needed is open acceptance, just as one feels lightness and weightlessness in a healthy body, the same feeling should extend to the finer and spiritual bodies of man too which also includes the mind. Though all religions are there for realizing one's infinite potentiality and divinity, they are actually proving to be a hindrance, cramping and narrowing one's perspective. As mentioned often in the 'Srimad Bhagavata' realized persons like Kapila, Kardama, Suka among many others "*went about the world with an expanded state of consciousness*", they harly speak nor act." Shyam: "what do you mean when you say that they hardly act, doesn't Lord Krishna in the Gita say that one should act and perform his (Karma) duty?" Agasthya: "Krishna also says that one should perform his duty without yearning for the fruits of his labor, that is, one should act without the feel that he is the creator, the doer, the achiever. Nor should he expect rewards for his labor and should be happy with whatever he gets. Moreover action is a must for the ordinary man, when realization dawns in him, there is nothing more to achieve nor attain. He realizes that he too is just part of the mega game of the Lord and like mentioned in many a holy text, he like the python doesn't even go in search of food, he consumes what comes by him once a while, that is, he eats only to nourish and nurture his body and mind and not very particular about it. Even breathing is considered an action(Karma)!"

Heidi: "Sir! But can one live without breathing?" Agasthya: "Of course one needs to breathe to live, but there are multiple sorts of breathing. Like explained deeply and profoundly by the Siddhar Thirumoolar in his masterpiece 'Thirumandiram' the 'art' of breathing itself is a deep science and he goes on to add that the one who masters the breath can even spurn 'Yama' the Lord of death. The common man takes four seconds for a single breath (4 seconds per breath = 15 per minute;900 per hour;21, 600 per day) while the dog and monkey breathe at a much faster pace the python's is much slower and the tortoise breathes only once every four minutes (hence lives for 600 years or so) and the 'Purna Yogi' or a full-blown Yogi breathes only once in 2.5 hours, so living for thousands of years is easy!

Heidi: "How would metabolism take place at such a slow rate of breathing?" Agasthya: "You must know that some species of bears like the brown bear of America and Polar bears go into hibernation during deep-winter season which is a sort of *suspended state of animation* when heart-beat as well as breathing is practically nil! Frogs, toads and some species of fish in Africa too survive for many years in such aforesaid states, in fact recently in the U.S. archeologists mistakenly broke a rock within which there was a live frog that had survived for billions of years according to carbon-dating but died in an instant due to the sudden climatic change! Moreover the Siddhars who are masters of the breath, breathe 'internally' which in Tamil is known as *'Ullh moochi'* whereby outside air isn't necessary, like the frog which can draw-in air through its skin they can draw-in air as well as nourishment through various means, so food, water, air *and* energy are always available to them! Even now there lives a person in Calcutta who hasn't consumed water or food for the past forty years. Doctors and scientists have conducted numerous trials and observations and find everything to be normal. He passes off only urine and says that he absorbs moisture from the air through his skin and nourishment from the sun's rays!"

Shyam: "You said earlier sir that even breathing is an action...?" Agasthya "Sri Rama in 'Rama Gita' has said: *"Thoughtless mind is Brahman"*, so literally for one to attain Brahman or God-Consciousness, one has to stop the flow of thoughts, which indeed is a very difficult thing to do. The mind and the breath are closely related, one can stop the mind (from functioning) by stopping the breath and vice versa when one gets control over the mind he can also by sheer will-power stop his breath! The exalted ecstatic-state of the Lord can be experienced here and now by stopping the mind, that is by entering into the state of 'no-mind' either by willfully stopping the breath or by attaining the 'Kevala Kumbaha'state (Perfect retention of breath in the Yogic-science) which happens on its own accord when in the deep state of meditation. In fact the Sufi Muslims would by sheer force of will hold their breath and fall faint in a state of ecstasy!

Heidi: "Sir! Do you mean to say that Yoga was also known to Islam and perhaps other religions of the world also?" Agasthya: "Yes of course! 'Yoga' was in Arabic known as 'Saluk', 'Pranayama' the art of control of the Pranic-force as 'Habs-e-dam' and even 'Nokku Varma Kalai' (in Tamil) the art of freezing or even killing another life-form by the power of sight alone as 'Habs-i-nazr'. Ancient Egypt and Greece (Pythagaros had learnt in mysticism schools in Egypt whose Pyramids have similar designs to ancient Indian Temples to awaken the 'Kundalini' the 'Cosmic Energy' also known as the 'Serpent-Fire' to both the cultures. Pythagaros in fact stayed in Egypt for 23 years and met Thales (one among the 'Seven Wise men' of Greece) as confirmed by Archimides) also had tenets of Yoga just to point out a few among the ancient civilizations. Yoga existed and exists in other 'worlds' also as Lord Krishna tells us in the Bhagavad Gita that He first taught the tenets of Yoga to the Sun (Sun god) and then to many others of this as well as other worlds through many countless 'Yugas'(eons). The ancient Chinese learnt the art of Yoga and meditation from the Buddhist monks of Tibet and thus 'Dhyan' or meditation became known as 'Chan' to the Chinese and it became known as 'Zen' to the Japanese, Korean as well as many other countries and spread all over the globe!

Shyam: "Sir, what about Judaism and Christianity? Did they who are the other two among the three 'Abrahamic Faiths' also know and practiced Yoga?" Agasthya: "The three main Jewish sects were: 'Essenes', 'Saducees' and 'Pharisees', and among these Jesus Christ was born among the 'Essenes' who had many aspects of Yoga and like the Indian 'Ashram' way of life and schooling, children were brought about by the society as a whole. In fact apart from the 'Torah', another very holy book of Judaism is the 'Kabala'(or Cabala, Kabhala) which is a very secretive book known to very few Rabbis even up to few centuries ago. The meaning of 'Kabala' in Jewish is "the shining frontal skull" and in 'Yoga' there is a breathing technique known as 'Kabala bheti'(bellows-like fast repetitive breathing) the practice of which also results in the frontal skull to glow in radiance (as a result of attaining Wisdom)!

It is a well known fact that almost nothing is known of the life of Jesus when he was between the ages of fifteen to thirty. He had travelled to the East, come to India and had been trained in the tenets of Yoga. The 'Magi' who had also travelled from the East and had been led to Bethlehem when Jesus was born were really 'Yogis' for whom 'Magic' and Supernatural Powers were second nature to them. Many ancient texts also mention that after Crucification, Jesus (who had not died on the cross as a Perfected Being can never ever be harmed nor killed) had lived on for well past ninety years in Kashmir. The late Swiss author and researcher 'Erik Von Daniken' in many of his books like 'According To Evidence' and 'Chariots of the Gods', provided even photographs of the tombs of Jesus Christ, Virgin Mary, Moses and of others in Kashmir India and in Pakistan also which all seem very controversial but are true!"

Heidi: "Doesn't 'Yogananda Paramahansa's' book 'The Autography of a Yogi' also has references to a meeting between 'Maha Avatar Babaji' and Jesus?" Agasthya: "Yes, it is said that Babaji had met Jesus and Adi Sankara and taught them 'Kriya Yoga' which is the 'internal breathing' I'd earlier told you about."

Shyam: "Sir, I've read and heard that You in fact are the Master and preceptor of Kriya Yoga, is that true?" Agasthya: "No! it was taught to me by the 'Adhi Guru' (First and Foremost Master, the Father) Lord Siva Himself!"

Heidi: "Sir, what about Lord Buddha's and the Buddhist tradition of 'Vipasana'?" Agasthya: "Unfortunately this wonderful 'Tantra' (technique) has been branded as Buddhist and therefore shunned by many. There is a wonderful 'Kashmiri Shaivism' (ancient Kashmiris who worshipped Lord Shiva as their Primal Lord) text 'Vijnana Bhairava Tantra' containing 112 tantras or techniques on how to directly experience the state of the Lord. The first nine among the 112 techniques deals on experiencing the exalted Infinite-State through aligning one's consciousness with the breath. There are also wonderful techniques provided by the ancient Tamil Siddhars to experience the Lord's state that also includes transcending the body and mind and thus experiencing the Infinite state of the Lord that of course makes one attain the 'Deathless-state' (*Sahakalai* in Tamil) immortality."

Heidi: "Sir, I thought Yoga can only extend one's life, but infinity …?"
Agasthya: "'Infinity' is already *programmed* within man! The Vedas clearly state that man was programmed to live for 100, 000 (hundred thousand) years in the first 'Yuga'(eon) known as 'Kreta yuga'(more than five million years ago), 10, 000 years in the second known as 'Treta yuga', 1000 years in the third known as 'Dwapara yuga' and a 100 years in the present one known as 'Kali yuga'. What is also true is that 'reprogramming' can be done in any of the yugas by practicing any of the various Yogas be it 'Bakti Yoga' (Devotion), 'Raja Yoga' (King of Yogas) or 'Jnana Yoga' (Wisdom). All Yogas ultimately leads one to Realization of the Self where he understands and experiences that he is an extension of the Supreme Self. There is absolutely no difference between the Self (Soul) and the Lord (as claimed by many Perfected Beings like Thirumoolar). In that state of Realization, one understands and experiences the claim of the Vedas that the Soul is 'Satchitananda' – 'Sat' – Existence Absolute;'Chit' Knowledge - Absolute;'Ananda' – Bliss Absolute. Moreover the Yogic texts say that among the 36 'tattvas' (Principle ingredients or concepts) that make a man, one is the *'Kala tattva'* or 'Time concept' and when one through Yogic-means transcends them, he even in the physical can live for eternity!"

Agasthya continued on man's eternity: "Lord Krishna in the Bhagavad Gita has explained the body to be a field of energy (*Kshetram*) which in the microcosmic-level in the contracted form is the human body but when the 'knower' of the field *(Kshetrajnan)* expands and in the macrocosmic-level could cover the entire universe. The 'Saiva Siddhanta' philosophy of the Tamils of India have clearly stated that 'change' or transformation happens in evolution from the lowest form of life possible to the highest which is man only until realization. After that evolution is not like milk being transformed into curd, but like the blossoming of a flower, not unlike a folded circus-tent which is small but when unfolded becomes immensely big ("*padalam kudil anar pola*")! You should understand that the Self the Soul extends to infinity and hence is not bound by either space and thus time. When one realizes that he is infinite, he is the Infinite! Only a full-blown Yogi like Thirumoolar and many others who with Absolute Faith had realized the infinite –state could claim: "*Siva and Jiva (the individual Soul) are no different; Jiva does not realize Siva; When Jiva realizes Siva; Jiva remains firmly entrenched as Siva."*

Heidi: "Sir, You were telling us about the 6000 births we take as humans alone, why don't we remember at least some of those births? Is there scientific basis and proof of such preceding births?" Agasthya: "For most people even remembering what they ate the previous day or the previous week would not be possible and recollecting experiences that had occurred before they were three or four years old would seem impossible. Moreover many experiences would not be pleasant and it'd be best to be forgotten and imagine the stress and turmoil that would be the outcome if 'Total Recall' of all activities of all previous births were possible. To prevent man from turning insane and provide him with opportunity to ascend further, the Lord out of mercy has put him under the spell of 'Maya' that is the illusive Power of the Lord. But Total Recall *is* possible, but for that to happen, one has to become a *'Trikala Jnani'* (literally Master of the three times – the past, present & future) and turn 'Perfect', a Purna Yogi, a Siddhar! When Lord Buddha attained enlightenment, he in a flash remembered 400 of his previous lives, the life of an eagle, a hare, a serpent, a deer ..! Saint Manickavasagar too (who lived in the 5ᵗʰ century A.D. in the Tamil Land) in his 'Thiruvasagam' cried out in pain after recollecting experiences of innumerable lives: *"From a blade of grass, to shrubs, plants, creepers, trees, serpents, ghosts, titans, man, angels, gods, yogis, hermits, everything, I've taken innumerable births and grown tired and weary in the process my Lord!"*

Agasthya continued: "You were asking me about scientific proof, though it is very difficult to prove scientifically prove these ultra-subtle experiences that the Soul undergoes that the Lord has for the good veiled from us, there have been some exceptions. Research has been going on all over the world for quite some time about people having recollections of their previous lives and all of them cannot be just wished away. There are countless claims of people remembering either their loved ones or people who had seriously harmed or even murdered them in their past lives. Many persons have correctly identified their killers and the hidden weapons while others have named the town, house and close family members in previous lives. Moreover Carl Jung the pupil of Sigmund Freud (the father of modern day psychology and psycho-analysis) explains that we have "*blocked-off memories*" of experiences gained through various lives starting from single-celled protozoa to plants, trees, birds, animals, man which are all passed on through our DNA! More than that common sense and deep thinking and analysis would bring us to the conclusion that just as a person to become a doctor, scientist, engineer or just about anything would need years and several stages of learning to gain that sort of higher-state, evolution and enlightenment would surely need billions of years and countless life-times to cross to gain experiences, learn and transcend further and finally turn Perfect!

Heidi: "Sir, You had told us about the 112 tantras or techniques mentioned in the 'Vijnana Bhairava Tantra' to help us experience the state of the Lord, can you explain to us a few simple but effective ones among them? Agasthya: "Apart from aligning one's consciousness with various forms of the breath, there is one which guides you to stand out in an open field filled with lots of trees, bushes and open space in a moon-lit night and blend in with the trees, rocks, shadows..! The idea is to expand one's consciousness and merge with infinite space, which though seems difficult is quite easy for that exactly is our true nature!"

Agasthya continued: "Another easy technique is also being taught by the Zen masters. One needs to visualize the surrounding air as if it were smoke or mist and while the master made a clapping-sound with the help of a clap-board, one should start to inhale while imagining that all goodness was being drawn in, at the next sound one should start to exhale while imagining that if at all any bad residues within were being rejected. Visualization helps greatly and during the rainy season, moisture-laden fine clouds could be seen floating around tree-tops, one can easily then inhale while imagining with faith that all the goodness of nature were being drawn in! This technique also greatly helps in flushing out toxins in the body of which the west is just beginning to acknowledge and more progressive and open thinkers accept that more than eighty percent of toxins can be flushed away through just proper breathing."

Shyam: "Sir, what is proper breathing? And how are we to correct it?" Agasthya: "Through proper breathing one ultimately turns 'Perfect' transcends space and time and turns eternally young. The new born baby's breathing-pattern is the one to be followed. If observed keenly one can see that the baby's stomach rises and falls and not the chest as many wrongly presume. The Japanese 'Samurai' warriors especially have mastered this art and know that when the chest is expanded in breathing it is known as 'Yo-ibuki' or hard-style breathing that is used during combat (and avoiding fatigue) and it is the opposite of in 'In-ibuki' during meditation-breathing, though both use the entire natural breathing apparatus unlike the modern-day norm which utilizes merely the top of the lungs.

Moreover the Yogic-texts say that the 'new' born baby's breath is Perfect for the new born baby's breath is said to be 12 inches long while ours measures 8 inches. Tirumoolar elaborates on this in his Thirumandiram 2546:

"At the tip of the nose is the breath, twelve finger-breath long, At the peak is the Sahasra Chakra, That verily is the Lord's abode; None know this; The Vedas that in expansiveness truths expound, of this was hesistant to speak; Such indeed is Lord's greatness."

We have a *tenth* opening at the crown of our head when we are born known as the *'brahmarandra'* in Sanskrit and *'brahma pugzai'* in Tamil (known to modern science as the 'anterior fontanelle') which literally means the doorway or portal of the Lord. The opening gets obliterated when we are around nine months old, until then it is soft and feels spongy to the touch. The tenth opening leads from a secret passage starting from the upper-palate of the mouth known as *'annakku'* or *'unnakku'* or 'inner-tounge' in Tamil, through which flows 'Prana' (air being only the outer manifestation that we breathe in while prana is the dynamic sum total of all forces in nature) flows. Prana flows through the secret chamber only in new born babies and in the Yogi (the Yogi also *leaves* his body through the tenth opening having predicted the exact moment of death many months or even years earlier) and hence the breath is twelve inches long. So we lose four inches of breath for every normal breath we inhale in, which again increases as we take on more strenuous work. When we breathe in prana through the mystical passage, we once again *turn* Perfect, we are no more bound by space or time, ambrosia or the elixir of youth flows which turns the person *eternally young* as the following song of Thirumoolar who was a Siddhar or Perfected-Being of the

Tamil Land (who lived for 3000 years) says in his Thirumandiram 805: *"If you can send the breath twain, into the internal-tounge's upper-cavity, You shall not be bound by time; And the gates of nectar will open be; Graying and wrinkling will disappear for all to see; Youthfull will the person be, This is the Word of the Lord Nandhi."*

Heidi: "Sir, you said that almost eighty percent of toxins within the body can be flushed out just by proper breathing! Can all diseases and toxins be wiped clean just through Yogic means?" Agasthya: "Not just diseases and toxins, but even deadly cuts, the effect of poisons and the ultra-subtle manifestations of 'Karma' can be cured and nullified through Yogic means! Almost all diseases are Karmaic in nature! The bad acts we'd committed (like un-wantonly killing various forms of life including that of mankind)in past lives manifest as what could be broadly termed as 'magnetic-impurities' in the subtle 'causal body' of man known as 'Kaarana udal' and/or 'Karu udal' – 'embryonic-body' in Tamil. The physical body or 'Annamaya kosa' (nourished mainly by food) is only the outer manifestation, there are four other subtle and ultra-subtle bodies: the 'Pranamaya kosa' or 'etheral body' (nourished by Prana), the 'Manomaya kosa' or 'mind body', the 'Vijnanamaya kosa' (which is the 'reasoning' or 'scientific body') and the 'Anandamaya kosa' or 'bliss body'. The Yogi or the Siddhar who is the Perfect One with the vision of the 'third eye' of Wisdom can *see* the magnetic-impurities that manifests in the causal body of man grossly as knots but minutely in the shape of deadly-looking miniscule bats, crabs, scorpions and spiders latched on with their sharp claws and hooks. The Yogi can see these cancerous knots in themselves *and* in others and in many ways can comb and sweep them away!"

Agasthya continued: "These magnetic impurities can be cleaned and eradicated by purification holy baths like bathing in salt-rich ocean-waters, through 'music-therapy' that is by treatment by the sounds of the vocal, drums, wind and string-instruments, chanting of prayers and mantras etcetera. Magnetic-field therapy, light-therapy and sweeping the body clock-wise with rock-salt, sun and moon-light bathing at specific times all prove extremely beneficial. The ancient Tamil Siddhar Thiruvalluvar in his 'Thirukural' has said: "Those who perform thavam (penance) create their

Karma (destiny)("*Thavam seyvaar thum karmam seyvaar...*"); all others wallow in pain and grief being ensnared in desires and cravings." Through 'Thavam' or penance all residues can be burnt and through meditation, one can see and visualize the harmful knots on the subtle bodies and sweep them away even before they manifest as deadly and sometimes fatal diseases in the physical body."

Agasthya: "When Dhurvasa (in 'Shiva Maha Purana')one of the greatest Yogis asked Lord Shiva Himself on how one could be absolved of all his sins (which are the reason for the manifestation of diseases), the Lord replied that even by performing one *Uttama Pranayama* ('Uttama' – foremost, pure, complete) the person would be absolved of all his sins. Pranayama is the art of controlling the flow of the Pranic –force within and without (the body) thereby Perfecting the entire body governed by 72, 000 '*nadis*' or astral nerves. Thirumoolar the great Master of Yoga and Siddhar explains that inhaling('Puraka') prana through the left-nostril(possessing the qualities of the moon)for16 'matras'(counts), retaining ('Kumbaka')(possessing qualities of 'Agni')for 64 matras, exhaling through right-nostril (qualities of the sun)for 32 matras is most ideal, performing it otherwise is most harmful. If you were wondering on how to time a 'matra' mentioned above, understand that slowly chanting of 'Siva Siva' once equals 4 matras, so inhaling should be done for a time of chanting 'Siva Siva' 4 times that equals 4 x 4 = 16 matras; retention should be done for chanting 'Siva Siva' 16 times that equals 16 x 4 = 64 matras; and exhalation for chanting 'Siva Siva' 8 times that equals 8 x 4 = 32 matras."

Heidi: "Sir, please explain to us how by inhaling and exhaling to certain specific timings and proportions one can gain such extraordinary benefits!" Agasthya: "You should understand that entire creation is nothing but matter and energy. And Prana known as 'Vasi' in Tamil is the Dynamic aspect of the Lord, many Siddhars have claimed: "*Vasiyum Isanum Ondru*" – "Vasi and the Lord are One and the same," also by reversing the word 'Vasi', turns out to be 'Siva' one among the thousand Holy Names of the Lord! Vasi or Prana is the ultra-subtle dynamic- energy present in air, while air is just the outer manifestation of Prana. Just as air contains 24 percent of oxygen which is vital to our survival, Prana the sum total of all forces in nature that includes electricity, magnetism, gravity everything is present in air that is extremely vital. There are 72, 000 nadis present in the body, among which 101 are important and among them 10 are most important, three very important and one the most vital nadi. The ten important nadis ones are: the left and right nostril nadis; left and right eye nadis; left and right ear nadis; tounge nadi; excretory and reproductive nadis; and finally the most vital one being the 'Sushumna' nadi that runs from the base of the spine, past the mystical cavity existing between the upper-palate of the mouth and the crown of the head. When through Yogic means Prana is made to rise through the Sushmna, the 'Kundalini' or the 'Cosmic-Energy' lying coiled in slumber at the 'Muladhara Chakra' at the base of the spine is awoken and gently made to rise along with Prana. There are six main chakras above the hip and the Kundalini force activates each of them as it ascends and when it finally flows into the seventh one above the cranium of the head known as the 'Sahasra Chakra', the person attains 'Superconsciousness' and becomes 'One' with the Lord!"

To the simultaneous questions on Kundalini and the Chakras put forth by both Shyam and Heidi, Agasthya answered: "The Chakras are 'vortexes' of energy-centres that exist (in the subtle bodies) over vital organs, hormonal glands and nerve-plexuses. Since they resemble colorful flowers and rotating discs they are known as Chakras. The chakras are also 'Wisdom-centres' and storehouses of knowledge that includes the 'tattvas' or principle ingredients of among others the 'Pancha boothas' (principles of the five basic elements in nature: earth, water, air, fire and space), the concepts of the 'seven upper worlds', and the sound-vibrations of 50 letters being the number of the Sanskrit alphabets, also of the ancient Tamil alphabets (before the 'round-lettered era' – 'vatta ellhuthu kalam') and which are also the vowel-consonants of the Japanese and Chinese language-alphabets(though the Chinese language has more than 50 to 60, 000 alphabets, 50 are its vowel-consonants).

The Kundalini is the Cosmic Energy utilized by the Lord during Creation. It is the Dynamic Energy and female aspect of the Lord while the Lord is the male and The Potential. It exists in its fiery-form within the core of the earth as well as within all the heavenly bodies. It also exists in human as well as all creatures that have back-bones. In man the kundalini lies coiled like a serpent (the ancient Egyptians knew it as the "Serpent of Fire") in slumber at the base of the spinal column at the Muladhara or base chakra. When aroused through Yogic-means it rises along with the Prana, slowly winds its way up and as it ascends, activates each of the chakras and when it finally flows into the Sahasra chakra at the crown of the head, the Union is Total, since the male and female aspects of the Lord (the 'Yin' and 'Yang' according to the Chinese) merge, He is the '*Shiva-Shakti Swarupa*'.

The person who has thus attained Super-consciousness is now is a 'Purna Yogi or a Full-blown Yogi to whom nothing is unknown! Since he transcends the tattvas or principle ingredients of the Pancha Boothas or five basic elements in nature, he becomes the Master of Nature. Having transcended the tattvas of 'the seven upper worlds' (and seven important Chakras below the waist that contain the tattvas of the 'seven lower worlds') he becomes Omniscient and could thus be anywhere through teleportation in space at a time. Having transcended the 50 letters that exists as fifty 'mantras' (potent sound-vibrations) distributed among the six chakras (the 'seed-vowels') that are again contained in the Five ('life-vowels') 'NA-MA-SI-VA-YA', he in an instant comes to know all world languages and their texts, and even the languages of the birds and beasts and also heavenly languages for the five 'life-vowels' contain the entire gamut of sounds that could be uttered by one and all!"

To the question of whether other religions too had stressed on the fact that man could attain the state of Perfection, Agasthya answered: "The Lord Jesus Christ in the Holy Bible, Matt.5, 48 says that one should attain the Perfect-state of the Lord. And again in Rom:8, 29 says that the '*eternal plan*' is to make everyone conform to the image of the son who himself is in the exact image (replica) of the Father." "Among Indian philosophies and religions, though there are many, six are considered primary. Among the six, 'Vaishnavism' considers Lord Vishnu as the Primary God and there is a very interesting narrative in the 'Ramayana' that too accepts that there is no difference between the individual soul and the Eternal Soul: When this question was put to Lord Rama, he answered that all world religions could be categorized under three philosophies and he directed Hanuman his devotee to provide the answer for he had *experienced* the three states - Hanuman replied: *"As long as Iam bound by the body and traces of cravings and limitations remain, You are the Lord and Iam a loyal servant; when Knowledge of the Soul (jivatmabodha) dawns in me, You are the Perfect-One (Purna) and Iam an exact- replica, an aspect (amsa)of You; when the Soul's Wisdom in its entirety which is Pure Consciousness (shuddha chaitanya bodha) shines in me, there is absolutely no difference between You and me, You are Me and Iam You."*

Heidi: "Sir, You had said that when man attains Super consciousness he in an instant comes to know all world languages *and* its texts! Can you be more specific?" Agasthya: "The late Carl Sagan as the Director of NASA and SETI (Search for Extraterrestrial Intelligence) in his book 'Contact' says that he chose the 50 letters of the Sanskrit alphabets to be inscribed on a golden record (so that radio-waves would not corrupt the messages) that also had many other relevant information about our civilization that was placed in 'Voyager' that was launched into space in 1967 for a chance encounter with alien intelligence. Carl says that he particularly chose the 50 letters of the Sanskrit alphabets for it was the most 'complete' language and they cover and contain all letters and all possible sounds (that is why the 50 letters that cover and contain all languages and sounds emanated are known as *'Mathurukatchara' – that which is the base to all languages*) and they also happened to be the vowel-consonants of the Japanese, Chinese language alphabets and the total Tamil alphabets which were existent before the 'round-letter era'(*vataelluthu kalam*).

Tirumoolar in his Thirumandiram: *"Fifty letters alone contain all Vedas; Fifty letters alone contain all Agamas; When source of fifty letters become revealed; Fifty letters become Five letters."* Although many Yogic texts explain on the distribution of the fifty letters as fifty sound-vibrations among the six chakras, Swami Sivananda's 'Kundalini Yoga' elaborates deeply on the subject. The full-blown Yogi not only comes to know all languages and their texts but becomes the Master of the '64 Arts' or the '64 branches of knowledge' that contain all worldly knowledge. There is now mention of 'Acquired Savant Syndrome' all over the world, whereby due to receiving un-expected blows to the head people have become instant geniuses in various fields. Some have started to speak in languages they had no contact with what so ever, some have become masters in music, mathematics and various other fields! But it is Yoga which very clearly says that all the arts and sciences are already programmed within us as the 'Kalai tattva' or the 'Art Principle' and they all are activated and recollected by the Yogi.

Shyam: "Sir, you had said something about re-programming, do you mean to say that 'genetic-engineering', 'gene-splicing' and 'DNA programming' was known to even the ancient Yogis?" Agasthya: "Yes! But you must understand that there have been countless cycles of advanced civilizations even here on earth that have been erased completely without any trace. Many lost cities and countries are even now being unraveled in China and the American continent buried under sand and time. Tiny, giant and what seem to be alien skeletons (of humans)are also being discovered. That there have been many previous cycles of creation in which man existed in a much different shape and size than what we now possess and that Adam is only the father of 'modern' or should we say 'present-day' man is mentioned by an Islamic scholar and holy man: The celebrated Shaikh, Muhyi-ud-Din al-'Arabi, regarding to the *insila* (a state of contemplation, when it is held the soul of man leaves the body and wanders about without regard to time or space), once when he was in the vicinity of the holy and revered Ka'ba (Caaba), it happened that, absorbed in mental reflections on the four great jurisconsults of Islamism, he 'saw' three very tall persons engaged in *'tawaf'* or circumambulating the holy Ka'ba and they were as tall as the revered structure (which is about 38 feet high). When he arrested them by the power of his sight (known as 'habs-i-nazr'), the leader pleaded with him to release them, and he told them that on the name of Allah the mercifull, he should tell him who they were, and he replied that they too were men who lived forty thousand years ago on earth. When the Shaikh asked him how that could be when it was only six thousand years since the advent of Adam, the stranger replied: ***The Adam you speak of was the father of the human race, and though since his time only six thousand years have elapsed, thirty other worlds preceded him.*** *In the Traditions of the Pride of all Beings (the Prophet), and the Sovereign ('Ali), it is said, ' Certainly*

God created the Adam (Man) you know of, **after the creation of an hundred thousand others**, *and I am one of those.*"

The Vedas say that during the beginning of a cycle of creation, "*the Creator created everything as they existed in the previous cycle.*" Moreover Tirumoolar says that he visioned countless cycles of creation and destruction "as equal in numbers as numerous grains of rice that boil over within a pot." In the 'Yoga Vashista' Vashista tells the young prince Lord Rama of meeting 'Kaka Busandha' a full-blown Yogi who lives in a secret cave north-east of Mount Kailash in the Himalayas who has been a witness to 7500 cycles of creation and destruction! When questioned on his longevity and his youthful-state, the Yogi said that he watched the 'gap' or interval between two breaths which helped him transcend space and time. Moreover to explain to you about time and its relativeness, I'll explain to you what the Vedas say about it: The Vedas say that Lord Brahma the Creator's one day-time is equal to 4.32 billion years of our earth-time; a night-time again equals another 4.32 billion years; at the end of every day-time for the Creator due to relentless heat and then rainfall everything is destroyed and life-forms take shelter in the Creator in the night-time and creation once again resumes during the day. After 100 such years for the Creator (8.64 billion years x 360 x 100 years) everything and all planets their satellites and stars of the three lower worlds are destroyed (after 100 years of deadly heat followed by 100 years of relentless rain) when all atoms and their sub-particles would explode and return back to their original self being 'Nada Bindu' or the 'Eternal Sound-Light' vibrations being the 'Basic Building Blocks' of Nature (imagine the deadly big bang that would be the outcome!)"

"Regarding DNA re-programming many Yogis and even the Lord Jesus Christ's Apostles had re-programming done for themselves!" Seeing the surprise and bewilderment on the faces of his guests Agasthya continued: "Do you know that a recent global study on AIDS conducted by WHO found to their surprise that the DNA of prostitutes of a particular African country had been 'naturally programmed' to be immune to the HIV virus just as the DNA of the mongoose is naturally programmed to be immune to the venom of snakes, even to that of cobra venom. There is a person in north India who is immune to all snake poisons and even that of potassium cyanide! When the Apostle Paul was bitten by a deadly viper in an island near the African continent, he was not at all affected by the deadly poison as was earlier prophesized by Christ himself. Jesus had also to the question put up by his disciples the apostles as to how were they to propagate his teachings all over the globe when they wouldn't know the various languages of different countries and regions, replied that the Holy Spirit would enter their tounges and they would come to know those languages, and it happened like that! Similarly when Lord Muruga wrote the words 'Aum' on the tounge of Saint Arunagirinathar and asked him to bring forth 'Pearls' (*"Mutthai tharu.."*), like when water flows gushes out in spate when the sluices of a dam are opened, words that were pearls of wisdom flowed out and thus was created the masterpiece 'Thirupugazh'. Saint Kumaraguruparar could immediately start to converse fluently in Urudu with a north Indian King in Benares just by praying to the Godess! Sadasiva Brahmendra just by touching the amputated portion of his own hand that was cut off by an enraged Badshah was able to in an instant transform it to its normal self! People had seen Chaitanya Prabhu and Saint Ramalingam 'turn' young and witness the transformation of their hair turning black and wrinkles on their skin vanish and turn youthfull!"

Heidi: "Sir, You had said that all diseases could be cured, can you say how many diseases are there?" Agasthya: "According to the Western Medicine System there are 3000 diseases and the ancient 'Ayurvedic' medicine system also confirms on that number. But the 'Siddha' Medicine system of the Southern part of India specifies that there are 4448 diseases. There are even references to AIDS which say that due to immoral sexual indulgence the physical body becomes barren and would turn out to be "life-less like a dead-tree".

Heidi: "Sir, can one recognize and identify a full-blown or Purna Yogi?" Agasthya: "It'd be next to impossible to identify such a person for they would keep a very low profile and humbly say that they knew next to nothing! The characteristics of such a person is explained the 'Srimad Bhagavatam' (in characteristics of the Lord's devotee; Bk.XI, Discourse II, Narada visits Vasudeva and reproduces the dialogue between King Janaka and the nine Yogiswaras) *"Hari said: 44) He is the foremost of the Lord's devotees who sees himself established in all cratures as in the Lord, and sees all creatures established in his own self as in the Divine Soul….*" And Lord Krishna Himself in the Bhagavad Gita says: "*To see me in all creatures is the highest form of spiritualism.*" When Saint Ramalingam claimed: "*Whenever I saw withered-crop, I too withered!*", it was just not sympathy he felt for the plant, but he practically *experienced empathy* for their state is such that when a plant, a tree or bird or animal experienced hunger or pain, he too experienced them and whenever a plant or animal was satiated and experienced happiness, he too experienced them!"

To the question on how that was possible, Agasthya replied: "While the normal person's mind and his consciousness is confined within the field that is his body, the Yogi's field is much more expanded. Even in normal times, that is when they are not meditating, their field of consciousness would be *several* miles in circumference hence all life-forms would be affected positively and come under *their* control.

One can certainly feel the peace and bliss in such a person's presence, the degree or quantum of peace cannot be measured or fathomed but the Holy Bible (Phil.4:7) addresses this quality as: "*the peace of god that surpasses all human understanding!*" Whenever Lord Rama or Lord Mahavira (though he was the 24th and final '*Thirthankara*' he was considered to be the founder of Jainism for he 're-established' it) entered a forest, birds, insects and wild animals would cry out in joy welcoming them. Flowers would bloom in the thousands, even if it were un-seasonal, fruits would ripen and hang in bunches. Friend and foe like the tiger and deer, frog and serpent would all stand together and cry out in unison. Grass would sprout wherever their blessed-feet went and even dead barren plants and trees would germinate and sprout-out new green shoots!" It is also well known that a charging wild elephant in musth calmed down and sat before Lord Buddha while his followers ran helter skelter! Many a saint like Thirunavukarassar and Prahalada were not affected even by deadly poison, fire or even by throwing them down steep cliffs! When Thirunavukarrasar was tied to a giant mill-stone and pushed into the depths of the ocean-waters, even the 'dead-stone' floated like a boat and carried him to shore, the place even now near Chennai on the coast of the Bay of Bengal is known as 'Thonivoor' or 'Boat Town'!"

To the question whether physical transformation and Transfiguration takes place during and after turning perfect, Agasthya replied: "Yes it does happen! Like Moses attained transfiguration and his face glowed after seeing God face to face on Mount Sinai, many a Yogi attained transfiguration and even took on the exact replica of the Lord and attained *"four arms and shoulders"* as mentioned often in the Srimad Bhagavatam and the Thiruvilayadal Puranam.

The prayers and mantras he chants protects him like when the Lord Jesus was about to be arrested by thirty soldiers of the Roman governor Pontius Pilate, they were flung back even as they neared him; and when robbers lobbed huge stones and boulders upon Saint Thyagaraja and the retinue that followed him, the missiles bounced back on the attackers without hurting the Saint's accomplices!

There are many states that a Yogi goes through, he attains for example the *'Kaarana Kaarya rupa'* (the 'Cause-effect body') whereby his body has a distinct form but is not within anyone's grasp! No weapon could hurt such a person as a sword, bullet or weapon would merely pass through him nor could his image be captured on film! The bullets of 750 rifles fired simultaneously by Armenian soldiers merely passed through the 'Bab' the founder of the 'Ba'hai' faith in 1845 in Iran. Though the ropes that tied the Bab to the stakes were found burnt, he could not be seen and later they found him conversing with his followers in an underground cell!

The image of Saint Ramalingam (as well as Lahiri Mahasaye the pupil of Yukteshwar who in turn was the pupil of Maha Avatar Babaji) could not be captured on film in the early 1870's though three attempts were made by professional photographers (with their box-cameras and tripods) brought in from Madras. What was even more surprising was only the Yogi's image was a blank though the images of all those around him were captured on film. Pouring incessant rain did not in the least affect or drench Saint Kumaraguruparar (of the 17th century A.D.) nor put off the flame of the lamp he held in his hands though he stood all night in the heavy downpour!

The Yogi also attains the *'Swarna deha'* that is the body of golden-radiance and finally attains the *'Jnana deha'* or the 'Wisdom-body' and he de-materializes like Mira, Andal, Saint Pattinathar and Saint Ramalingam did and some times even before the presence of hundreds of onlookers like the first two did!"

Heidi: "Sir! Can you tell us what are the *basic building blocks* of nature, the elusive 'elementary particles', that even great scientists and astro-phycisits like Stephen Hawking have no answer to for in 'A Brief History of Time' Hawking says that since there are six varieties of 'quarks' they could be even further split?" Agasthya: "As you must know even the atom cannot be seen with the naked eye, and when they are further split, the electrons, protons and neutrons and even further, the quarks get illusively smaller! In fact 'Nada Bindu' ('Nadha Vindhu' in Tamil) the 'Eternal Sound-Light Vibrations' are the basic building blocks of nature. The Vedas clearly state that at the end of the 'Maha Pralaya' or the great annihilation all atoms and their split-particles known as the 'parama anu' of the three lower worlds among the seven upper worlds would all blow up (after a hundred years of deadly drought followed by hundred years of relentless rain) and revert back to their previous original self 'Nada Bindu'."

Heidi: "Sir, can you please expand further on Nada Bindu?" Agasthya: "Nada Bindu *is* none other than the Formless Form of the Lord! It is from Nada Bindu the eternal Sound-Light vibrations that the primal sound 'Aum' originated and in fact it is the subtle-body of Aum and everything else expanded from the Line and Dot, the former symbolizes Sound and the latterLight."

To the question of Heidi on how would one function when the mind is destroyed, Agasthya replied: "The mind itself has four divisions: manas (mind or lower mind); chitta (will); buddhi (intelligence) and ahankara (ego). One needs to rise from the lower-mind that is centred in the medulla oblongata known as the 'animal brain' which governs most vital in-voluntary functions like breathing and heart-beat that is common to man as well as animals. The Yogi knows that only during fast and shallow breathing the orders are passed on from the reptilian or animal brain, but when in higher states of meditation and when the breathing drastically slows down, the orders originate from the higher reaches of the brain. Even modern doctors and hear-surgeons know only that minute electric-impulses originate from the brain to stimulate heart-beat, but the Yogi knows and realizes the truth and thus by transcending further up goes to the 'Nada Bindu' which *is* the Source and is able to even stop his heart-beat and breathing indefinitely!"

Shyam: "Sir, there seems to be no single and definite reply to the question as to from where does the soul activate the body, while some like the Japanese Zen masters say that the navel-chakra (the manipura chakra) is the Core ot the Centre, others say it is the eyebrow-centre (the ajna-chakra) is the Core! Which really is the Centre?" Agasthya: "The Zen masters have also said: "The mind is no where in particular!" Great Siddhars actually say that the Star, the Soul exists twelve inches *above* the crown of the head. Thirumoolar's Thirumandiram delves seeply into this subject, it says that when the soul activates the body utilizing all the physical and subtle-body tattvas or instruments at the eyebrow or 'third-eye' centre the state is known as 'Jagra' – the 'woken-state'(that is why in Tamil when one is advised to be fully conscious, carefull or attentive the word 'Jagrathai' is used); when the soul descends to the throat-centre after losing some of the instruments it is known as 'Swapna' – the 'dream-state'; after descending to the heart-centre after losing some more instruments it is known as the 'Sushupti' state; when it descends even further and resides purely alone in its splendor, it is known as 'Turiya'. During deep meditation, there is also ascendency and during such a journey when the soul with total awareness is taken to the crown of the head, the state is also known as 'Turiya', but the Siddhars ascend even further twelve inches above the crown of the head and that state is known as 'Turiyatita' where the person becomes a 'Purna Yogi' or a 'Fullblown-Yogi' who is no different from the Lord!"

Heidi: "Sir! Like Albert Einstein was also able to explain to the lay-man in simple words his theory of relativity, can you explain this in simple words?" Agasthya: "When you say for example the President of the United States rules from Washington D.C., what is actually meant is his power, focus, care and attention extends to all the states, its boundaries and every nook and corner of the country. Likewise the soul governs the entire body, when one aligns with the soul and regains soul-consciousness, joy and bliss being one of its qualities is felt even at the end of every finger and toe-tip(even the hair-ends) and in that state disease and ageing finds no place while youth and tremendous vigour is the order of the day!"

Shyam: "Sir, how is to one meditate daily while living and leading a normal life?" Agasthya: "You need to delve often into the state of *no-mind* which actually means that you and the Lord are in the same wave-length and the 'Rama Gita' in particular says: "*Thoughtless mind is Brahman*". That would finally lead you to be *always* in that state. It is often mentioned in many texts like the Srimad Bhagavata that great Yogis and Siddhars like Kapila and Kardama went about the world "*with an expanded state of conscuiusness*". The Lord Jesus Christ too says in the Holy Bible that "the apostle knows more about you than what you know about yourself" – this is absolutely true for in an expanded state of consciousness the apostle exists within everyone and hence reading their thoughts or gaining their knowledge in their entirety is entirely possible! What it also means is that all life-forms in the immediate vicinity are positively influenced and there is no fear or enimity and only joy and vitality is experienced by one and all! Unlike ordinary folk the Yogi knows and experiences the true nature of the Soul which *is* omnipresence. When one is in that state infinite things are possible for he *is* infinite! The physical body too begins to acquire the qualities of the subtle bodies as well as that of the soul just as one progresses in Yoga the physical body starts to levitate which in Sanskrit is known as *Uthapena,* similarly being in one or two distant places at the same time (teleportation) also happens! Just as the Yogic-texts say, the late Thiruvaroor Rathinasabapathy Pillai has in his 'Thiruvasagamum Sivarajayogamum' said that when one consciously transcends and crosses the 'Space-body barrier' which is a ultra-subtle barrier that exists twelve inches above the crown of the head and all around the body (known as *'Anda-Kosa yellai'* in Tamil), he is no more bound by Space and Time! The Lord too in the Shiva Gita says that the person who meditates with the *bhava* (feel, belief and faith) that he *is* the Lord in the expansive omnipresent-state is the most favorite to Him! What more one needs to say!"

Saying this the holy Seer Agasthya smilingly vanished into thin space and both Shyam and Heidi descended down the Pothigai Mountain with joy brimming in their hearts and went on with lightness in their step knowing that they were the very lucky and fortunate among billions who by coming into close proximity of the Divine (just as fluffs of cotton would burn when coming into contact with fire)had transcended beyond the "*pair of opposites*" for whom gold and stone were on the same league who did not differentiate between good and bad nor beauty and ugly - the state of equanimity that Lord Krishna emphasizes in the Bhagavad Gita and who *experienced* liberation then and there!

Ashtanga Yoga (Eight-limbed Yoga)

Although there are many Yogas, four are considered to be the most important ones – 'Bhakti' or the Yoga of Devotion, 'Karma Yoga' which is living a life of Dharma or Righteousness and performing one's duties without yearning for the fruits of one's labors, 'Hatha Yoga' is performing extreme body and mind purifying exercises and finally 'Raja' or 'Kundalini Yoga' which as the name itself is the 'King' among Yogas as it helps one surely attain both Wisdom (Jnana) and liberation (mukti). Raja Yoga is the safest and surest way to attain Super-consciousness or God-consciousness, though all Yogas ultimately yield the same result the Yogin (is the beginner while the Yogi is an accomplished one) practices a combination of all Yogas (which Sri Aurobindo had rightly named them as 'Integral Yoga')for ultimately without devotion towards God, Yoga becomes meaningless and Wisdom which is Divine-Knowledge otherwise known as enlightenment and God are one and the same.

Thirumoolar a full-blown Yogi who lived for 3000 years and created 3000 and odd songs in the Tamil land in his masterpiece 'Thirumandiram' says that one should be decisive in choosing Ashtanga Yoga by following which one could attain absolute knowledge and get deliverance from the misery-filled endless cycle of birth and death; Thirumandiram 551:

"Waver not this way and that,
follow the way of the eight-limbed Yoga, and reach Samadhi-state;
they who tread the blessed path, shall reach Jnana's peak;
no more are they in this vile-flesh born."

Man evolves over thousands of births right from the lowest form of life possible through the life of grass, shrubs, creepers, plants, trees, birds, animals, man to the enlightened and Divine Being. By attaining the Samadhi-state after the mind has been absolutely stilled, the seeker and the Object are one and only then does the misery-filled endless cycle of death and birth end.

Yoga had descended from Ultimate Heaven 'Kailash' or the 'Seventh' Heaven the realm of the Primal Lord Shiva and eight were the masters with Patanjali to profess in the northern land through his 'Yoga Sutras' in Sanskrit and Thirumoolar through his Thirumandiram in Tamil; Thirumandiram

Although most people know Yoga only through 'Yoga Asanas' which seem to be just physical exercises, in fact they prove to be more than just providing a supple and strong physical body.In fact many Yogi's say that only the first three aspects of Yoga (iyama, niyama and asana) are related to the physical while the rest (pranayama, pratyahara, dharana, dhyana, Samadhi) are related to the spiritual. But in reality the physical and spiritual act in tandem for though the physical body seem to be the base, it is actually from the finer or spiritual body (which in Tamil is known as the 'kaarana udal' or 'causal body';'Karu udal' 'embryonic-body')that the 'effect'('kaarya' in Tamil) that is the physical body takes shape.

Only with a strong, steady and firm seat can the mind be stilled whereby one's true nature which is divinity is realized. Saint Patanjali has right in the first of his 195 'Yoga Sutras' emphasized on this point by saying: "*Yoga chitta vritti nirodhaha*" – "Yoga is keeping the mind in an unchanged (tranquil) state". Lord Rama too in the 'Rama Gita' has said: "Thoughtless mind is Brahman (God)".The latter day Zen masters too of the east, particularly Japan to whom this knowledge of Yoga was passed on to by the Buddhist monks of Tibet had greatly valued and sought after the state of 'no mind' known as 'Mushin' in Japanese.

The eight limbs of Yoga are:
Iyama, Niyama, Asana, Pranayama, Pratyahara, Dharana, Dhyana & Samadhi. Each step prepares one for the next step and finally Samadhi is attained, the state where there is absolutely no difference between subject and object, the merger is complete, Thirumandiram 554:

"Iyama, niyama and countless asanas,
pranayama wholesome and pratyahara alike,
dharana, dhyana and samdhi to triumph
– these eight are the steely limbs of yoga."

Iyama
Iyama consists of ten do's and dont's: non-killing, non-lying, non-drinking,
non-lusting. Marked virtues are: being good, being just, sharing the good
things of life with others and knowing no blemish; Thirumandiram 555:

"He does not kill, does not lie, does not steal;
of marked virtues is he; good, meek and just;
He shares his joys, knows no blemish, neither drinks or lusts
– this the man who in iyama's way stands."

Niyama
Niyama;, Thirumandiram 556:
"Purity, compassion, frugal food and patience,
forthrighteness, truth and steadfastness
– these he ardently cherishes; killing, stealing and lusting he abhors
– thus stands with virtues ten, the one who niyama's way observes."
Further ten attributes of niyama; Thirumandiram 557:
"Tapas, meditation, serenity and holiness, charity,
vows in Saiva-way and Siddhanta learning,
Sacrifice, Siva puja and pure thoughts
– with these ten, the one in niyama perfects his way."

Asanas
Asanas which means 'seat' are postures and are said to be 84, 00, 000 in
number and among them 84 are said to be important and eight among them
very important; Thirumandiram 563:
"Bhadra, gomukha, padma and simha,
sothira, veera, and sukha,
these seven along with eminent svastika constitute the eight,
eighty and hundred, however, are asanas all in reckoned."

The above mentioned eight asanas are the most important. Asanas are not mere body postures, for they help in moulding the body into a strong, supple and efficient instrument. Regular practice of asanas is a must because they help a person to sit in a comfortable posture for extended periods of time without any feeling of discomfort. As a person progresses in Yoga, be it in asana, pranayama, pratyahara, dhyana or Samadhi gradually the passage of time is not noticed, so asanas prove to be of great help. Various asanas also help to be 'acu-pressures' that help to massage and pressurize vital nerve-plexuses and hormonal-glands to secrete vital juices and enzymes to help the body function in an efficient manner. And last but not the least, an erect bearing that is achieved only when the stomach, core and back muscles are strong and the spine is kept supple and at the same time straight, does the Kundalini energy which is the 'Creative' Power of the Lord rise (from its slumber at the muladhara chakra at the base of the spinal column) on its own accord when the necessary degree of evolvement is achieved. For Wisdom to blossom in man the Kundalini which is the dynamic energy of the Lord has to rise. It has to slowly wind its way upward and on its journey activate the other six vital chakras that are all 'Wisdom' and 'psychic-centres', finally flow into the seventh and most important 'Sahasra' or 'thousand-petalled' flower at the cranium of the head, rise even further up and merge with the 'Holy-Feet' of the Lord which is the 'Nada Bindu', the eternal sound-light vibrations and thus become the 'Source' of Wisdom.

Pranayama
'Prana' is the sum total of all forces in nature that manifests multi-universally and not just the air we inhale or mere oxygen as it is wrongly believed to be. The air is only the outer body that encloses within the dynamic prana. Prana is won over by practicing Pranayayama which is the process by which prana is controlled by regulation of breath. The vital, dynamic, 'sukshma' or subtle, fine and un-seen force of which breath is the outward manifestation can be gained control by exercising control of the gross breath. And since the mind cannot operate without prana, control of prana means control of mind, it is as simple as that! All forms of energy like heat, light, electricity, magnetism are all manifestations of prana. By controlling prana, the mind is controlled, through the mind the Will is won over, through the Will the individual Soul and hence the Supreme and he are One.

The seat of prana is the heart-region, prana is one but it has various functions in the human body and hence assumes five names which are 'prana', 'apana', 'samana', 'udhana' and 'vyana'. There are also five 'sub-pranas', they are 'naga', 'kurma', 'kirikara', 'devadatta' and 'dhananjaya'.Totally they are known as the 'dasa vayus' or 'ten vital vacuum-forces'. Description and functions of the ten vital vacuum-forces:

1. Prana:color – yellow; location – anahata or heart-chakra; function – respiration
2. Apana:color – orange; location – muladhara or in-between excretory organs; function – urine and faeces ejection.
3. Samana:color – green; location – manipura or nave-chakra; function – digestion.
4. Udana:color – violet; location – visuddha or throat-chakra; function – swallowing.Takes the soul to the crown of the head in sleep, separates the the physical from the astral body at death.
5. Vyana:color – pink; location – swadishtan that acts on the entire body; function – circulation of blood.

Sub-pranas:
1.Naga – causes belching and hiccoughs. 2.Kurma – causes opening and blinking of eye-lids. 3.Kirikara – induces hunger and thirst. 4.Devadatta – causes yawning. 5.Dhananjaya – causes de-composition of body after death.

Breath directed by thought under the control of Will is a vitalizing, regenerating force which can be utilized consciously for self-development, for healing many incurable diseases and for many other unimaginable purposes. Ninjas and Tanjians (very secretive Japanese and Chinese martial art exponents who developed tremendous physical and psychic powers and were utilized mainly used to protect Shoguns and Kings, who knew a "thousand ways and means" to assassinate people) by sheer will-power could send endorphins coursing through their blood-stream to severely injured portions in their bodies and cure for example deep sword cut-wounds in a matter of minutes that would normally take weeks or even months to cure!

Sadasiva Brahmendra a full-blown Yogi who lived more than three centuries ago in the Tamil land, once all of a sudden walked into the zenana of a badshah stark naked, the enraged badshah drew his sword and promptly chopped off his arm.The Yogi went away with a laugh and was duly followed by the king carrying along the severed arm.Sensing the presence of a divine person the king hurried after him to beg forgiveness but could catch up with the Yogi only after a couple of hours for such was the rapid pace set by him. After the king fell at the Yogi's feet and offered back the severed limb, the Yogi gestured king to place the severed limb at the wound-juncture, and by merely touching the mutilated limb, restored it back to its normal self which was as good as new!

Many Yogis had made even cancerous-growths disappear in a jiffy by merely touching them with holy ash. Hatha Yogis consider that Prana 'taatva' (element) is superior to manas (mind) tattva because prana is present even when mind is absent during deep-sleep, but actually in the state of no-mind, that is in the state of Samadhi, there is no prana also, that is even breathing stops.

By controlling the little waves of prana working through the mind, one could control the universal prana, so one could not even imagine the infinite power that would be available to such a person. Moreover when the prana tattva is conquered, the Kundalini energy being the Creative Power of the Lord too rises on its own accord, activates the other six chakras which all in turn contain the tattvas of the 'Pancha Boothas' or five basic elements in nature – earth, water, fire, air, space and when one transcends these, entire nature comes under his command. He would thus like Moses, Narada, Jesus Christ, Sage Vyasa, Prophet Mohammed, Raghavendra, Ramalingam, Adi Sankara, the Mother of Pondicherry, Aurobindo and hosts of others be able to have command over entire nature. Saint Thirunavukarasar was placed in a burning lime-pit, but he sang pleasantly that it was as cool as the evening river-side breeze! He was once again cast into the depths of the ocean-waters after being bound to a heavy mill-stone, but he along with the mill-stone floated to the sea-shore near Chennai to a place even now known as 'thoniyur' or 'boat village'!

Raging fire did not in the least affect Sita or Hanuman. The deep waters of the Indian Ocean parted to give way to Ayya Vaikuntar (just as the Red Sea waters gave way to Moses) who entered the ocean depths in Kanyakumari (Cape Comorin), closed after him and the waters of the Bay of Bengal many miles to the north parted again three days later when the Saint once again appeared, but as the Divine! Swami Sankarananda the disciple of Sivananda of Vadakara Kerala was able to stop a train at Shenkottai (during the British rule) and nothing could be made to move it until the Swami had taken his seat! Sankarananda's disciple Nityananda was not in the least affected after being compelled to consume deadly poison, but instead the person who forced him to quaff it coughed out blood and fell to his death! When as a young lad Saint Kumaraguruparar was left holding a lamp out in the open by his master and rain fell down in torrents the entire night, though everything in the vicinity was drenched, not a drop of water touched either the Saint or the flaming lamp as he was protected by the natural elements! The Mother of Pondicherry even as a child could calm down a deadly storm (by 'conversing' with the Spirit of the storm just as Jesus had done) which was threatening to capsize the ship that she along with others were travelling in Europe during early twentieth century. When robbers hurled down stones and rocks on the entourage of Saint Thyagaraja, the stones bounced back on the miscreants just as Pontius Pilate's soldiers were flung back when they at first went to arrest the Lord to crucify him!

Prana is the over-coat of the mind and if one can control prana, one can control the mind and 'Veerya' or 'Ojus' (the seminal power or energy) because they are all inter-related. Like the nervous system in the physical body, there is also one in the astral body. The prana in the physical body's of the gross aspect is known as the *'sthula prana'* which is the outward manifestation of prana while the one in the astral body being a subtle manifestation of prana is known as *'sukshma prana'*. But there is an intimate connection between the two pranas and inter-action between them.

By controlling breathing, one can consciously and efficiently control all functions in the body.Psychic cure, distant-cure, telepathy, television (visioning distant scenes of the past, present and future along with experiencing sounds known as *'trikala jnana'* or "Wisdom of the three times") as Nostradamus, Sage Valmiki (for Valmiki wrote the epic Ramayana *before* the incidents happened), Prophet Mohammed and Swami Vaikuntar, who both like many others visioned the process of creation as well as future events and gained many other 'siddhis' which are psychic and supernatural powers which are the effects of the control of prana.

One might wonder as how people like Nostradamus who was neither a divine-being or a Yogi could have gained or acquired such powers as many people around the world 'naturally' possess various psychic as well as 'Extra Sensory Perceptive Powers', clairvoyance, levitation tendencies etc. To this question, Lord Krishna in the 'Bhagavad Gita' tells Arjuna the warrior-prince that nothing is gained by chance and that knowledge gained in previous lives are never lost and are passed on over countless lives.

Moreover even if a Yogi stops his endeavors mid-way, nothing would be lost, he would in his next life be born again in a wealthy or in the midst of like-minded educated family in a conducive atmosphere and continue from the exalted place he had attained in his previous life. In fact the effect of all acts good or bad committed in previous lives are passed on in ultra-subtle form known as 'karma' which may manifest as mental or physical diseases or bring about poverty or riches, despair or hope, sorrows or joy. The Yogi or Siddhar (who is the Perfected Being) who has the sight of the 'third-eye' can actually see diseases manifesting over particular organs or parts of the physical body in the 'causal' body itself.

Printed in the United States
By Bookmasters